OPERATIVE LAPAROSCOPY

OPERATIVE LAPAROSCOPY

Maurice-Antoine Bruhat, Gérard Mage, Jean-Luc Pouly

Hubert Manhes, Michel Canis, Arnaud Wattiez

Translated by

Roger Duvivier and Thierry G. Vancaillie

McGRAW-HILL, INC
Health Professions Division

New York St. Louis San Francisco Aukland Bogotá
Caracas Lisbon London Madrid Mexico Milan
Montreal New Delhi Paris San Juan
Singapore Sydney Tokyo Toronto

OPERATIVE LAPAROSCOPY

1234567890   987654321

ISBN 0-07-008587-0

This book was set in Times Roman by Datapage International Limited.
The editors were Jane E. Pennington and Muza Navrozov;
the production supervisor was Richard Ruzycka.
Soulisse & Cassegrain was printer and binder.

Library of Congress Cataloging-in-Publication Data

Coelioscopie opératoire. English.
    Operative laparoscopy / Maurice-Antoine Bruhat . . . [et al.];
translated by Roger Duvivier and Thierry G. Vancaillie.
        p. cm.
    Translation of: Coelioscopie opératoire.
    Includes bibliographical references and index.
    ISBN 0-07-008587-0
    1. Laparoscopic surgery. 2. Generative organs, Female--Endoscopic surgery. I. Bruhat, M. A. (Maurice Antoine) II. Title.
    [DNLM: 1. Genital Diseases, Female--surgery. 2. Laser Surgery.
3. Peritoneoscopy.   WP 660 C672]
RG104.7.C6413 1992
618.1′45--dc20
DNLM/DLC
for Library of Congress   91-4893
                                                            CIP

Operative Laparoscopy. Translated from the original French edition entitled *Cœlioscopie Opératoire* by Maurice-Antoine Bruhat, Gérard Mage, Jean-Luc Pouly, Hubert Manhes, Michel Canis, and Arnaud Wattiez, published by MEDSI/McGraw-Hill, Healthcare Group, Paris, France, 1989.

Authors

Maurice-Antoine Bruhat, Professeur de Gynécologie, Polyclinique Gynécologie-Obstétrique, Médecine de la Reproduction, Université de Clermont-
Ferrand.

Michel Canis, Assistant des Hôpitaux, Chef de Clinique des Universités,
Polyclinique Gynécologie-Obstétrique, Médecine de la Reproduction, Clermont-Ferrand.

Gérard Mage, Praticien Hospitalier, Polyclinique Gynécologie-Obstétrique,
Médecine de la Reproduction, Unité de Chirurgie, Clermont-Ferrand.

Hubert Manhes, Attaché en Premier des Hôpitaux, Polyclinique Gynécologie-
Obstétrique, Médecine de la Reproduction, Clermont-Ferrand.

Jean-Luc Pouly, Praticien Hospitalier, Polyclinique Gynécologie-Obstétrique,
Médecine de la Reproduction, Unité de Fécondation médicalement assistée,
Clermont-Ferrand.

Arnaud Wattiez, Assistant des Hôpitaux, Chef de Clinique des Universités,
Polyclinique Gynécologie-Obstétrique, Médecine de la Reproduction, Clermont-Ferrand.

Translators

Roger Duvivier, M.D., Director of Gynecology, Winthrop University Hospital, Mineola, New York, and Assistant Professor of Obstetrics and Gynecology,
State University of New York at Stonybrook, New York.

Thierry G. Vancaillie, M.D., Director of the Center for Gynecologic Endosurgery; Clinical Assistant Professor in Obstetrics and Gynecology, University
of Texas, San Antonio, Texas.

Acknowledgments

We would like to acknowledge participation of Pierre Schoeffler, Claude Henry, Jean Bouquet de Jolinière, Guillaume Le Bouëdec, and Jean-François Ropert. We also appreciate the involvement of the faculty and resident staff of the C.H.U. of Clermont Ferrand and of other universities who have assisted us.

We express our sincere thanks to Martine Sbizzera and Christine Detruy for their dedicated participation in editing this manuscript.

For their daily untiring devotion, we extend our gratitude to the nursing staff under the direction of Bernadette Claustre and Reine Guerry Surveillantes.

To Raoul Palmer

Table of contents

Preface

Endosurgical drainage of pyosalpinx in 1971, excision of an ectopic pregnancy in 1972, channeling of a laser beam through an endoscope in 1977—it was certainly hard to imagine then that only a few years later laparoscopic surgery would go through the rapid developments and advances described in this book.

High hopes do little to ensure future success, but our earlier accomplishments helped us to persevere:

– Hubert Manhes and I created around us a cadre of young people who were eager to learn, anxious to search for new ways, to achieve, to convince, and to initiate the timid, yet true to the belief that it is our patients who are the ultimate beneficiaries of "genuine progress" and that the only real failure is mediocrity.

– Natives of a very old French province, we conceived new techniques that were to be disseminated to all other countries, including those that are technologically the most developed.

– We succeeded in preserving the recommendation of one of the greatest of our compatriots, Blaise Pascal, not to abandon *l'esprit de finesse* in favor of *l'esprit de géométrie*.

In our constant search for the refinement of endosurgical techniques and our quest for new instruments, we have always obeyed the basic principles that govern all progress in surgery: (1) surgical gentleness and elegance, (2) efficiency, and (3) cost-effectiveness.

Surgical gentleness and elegance

Surgical gentleness means an operative technique that minimizes tissue trauma, resulting in rapid return of the treated organ to normal physiology. What can be called an antiphysiologic act par excellence, the opening of the abdominal wall at laparotomy, is avoided; thus the peritoneum is spared the trauma of lap pads and retractors and contamination from the air.

Endosurgery is indeed minimally invasive. Pneumoperitoneum with CO_2 or other gases replaces lap pads; the Trendelenburg position functions as retractors. The magnification achieved with an endoscope leads to a surgical precision which approaches that of microsurgery. The lesions, and only the lesions, are treated, while surrounding tissues are all spared; indeed, herein lies the promise of CO_2 laser vaporization of endometrial implants in the surgical treatment of endometriosis; of a carefully executed intra-abdominal ovarian cystectomy; of the aspiration-evacuation of an ectopic pregnancy through linear salpingotomy.

New surgical techniques rely on basic physiologic principles and aim at reestablishing normal functions without recourse to traditional surgical techniques. A salpingotomy incision usually heals spontaneously, without sutures, and the tube recovers normal function. Using the CO_2 laser to evert the cuff of a neosalpingostomy avoids the trauma of suturing; fibrin glue facilitates the closure of a gaping ovarian incision or of a peritoneal defect.

Efficiency

Measured in terms of the ablation of lesions, functional recovery, and achievement of pregnancy, the results of endosurgery are identical to those obtained with open surgery.

Endosurgery is subject to rigorous evaluation of the lesions, which is not always the case in classic surgery. This evaluation shows us (as if it were necessary) that the results obtained are related to the extent of the lesions (e.g., in endometriosis) or to the degree of tissue destruction (e.g., in reconstructive surgery of the tube). Most important, endosurgery promotes a totally new therapeutic approach in which diagnosis, therapy, and prognosis are achieved simultaneously instead of consecutively. This calls for extreme care on behalf of the operator and for additional support by modern technology such as computer science.

Cost-effectiveness

Reduced morbidity

Endosurgery is not dangerous, as some might erroneously believe, but it requires special training of both the surgeon and the anesthesiologist and, above all, close collaboration between them.

Reduced discomfort for the patient

Avoiding the opening of the abdominal wall alleviates postoperative pain and allows for a rapid recovery of bowel function.

Reduced surgical trauma

Less aggressive manipulation of organs leads to a better prognosis, both short- and long-term. Endosurgery calls for gentler handling of structures than does open surgery.

Reduced cost

Endosurgery results in a shorter hospital stay and convalescence than does open surgery, resulting in a reduction in cost.

This book is not intended to be merely a manual of surgical techniques. Endosurgery has forced us to view gynecologic pathology in a different light.

First a diagnostic procedure, then a mode of access for surgical correction, laparoscopy has, in a natural progression, become the tool par excellence for drawing up the therapeutic plan—the most important step in the treatment of a disease.

A clear demonstration of this global approach is the evolution in our management of ectopic pregnancy since 1973. Early detection of tubal pregnancies led us to evacuate small hematosalpinges by endosurgical salpingotomy. It soon became evident to us that the tube heals rapidly and well without sutures. The size and site of some ectopic pregnancies caused us to define relative or absolute contraindications to endosurgery. We soon realized that persistent ectopic pregnancy or failed endosurgical management could be detected by monitoring hCG levels. The excellent fertility rate of our patients after ectopic pregnancy prompted us to develop an "ectopic score," which is highly predictive of the chances for subsequent pregnancy and of the risks of another ectopic pregnancy or of permanent infertility. Therefore, selection of either conservative or radical treatment with subsequent in vitro fertilization becomes possible. The above example clearly illustrates how the triad—diagnosis, therapeutic plan, and treatment—is an inherent part of any laparoscopy. Not only is it the goal, but it also is the obligation of all modern endoscopic procedures.

The first part of this book describes the basis for our endosurgical approach, along with its special requirements for anesthesia, specialized instrumentation, and rigorous surgical discipline and training. Thereafter, each chapter defines a particular problem and outlines the operative techniques, the results, the indications and contraindications. Throughout, the emphasis is placed on discussion of the critical role endosurgery plays in the treatment of such conditions as PID or ovarian cysts.

For the English-language version of *Operative Laparoscopy*, two chapters have been added which do not appear in the original French edition. We have taken advantage of the opportunity occasioned by this new printing to include the latest information on laparoscopic hysterectomy and laparoscopic lymphadenectomy.

This book condenses 15 years of our experience in operative laparoscopy, and it is illustrated with a selection of some 200 pictures out of thousands of slides.

We hope the reading of these pages will enthrall the reader as much as writing them has excited us.

We are certain this book will whet everyone's appetite for endosurgery and encourage further education and training in these techniques.

In conclusion, endosurgery is a faithful expression of the French school of thought, where respect for organ function and trust in physiologic repair of tissues go along with careful preoperative planning and creative utilization of all available resources to produce surgery that is efficient, elegant, and cost-effective.

M. A. Bruhat
Professor of Gynecology

1

Anatomy

Laparoscopy is a surgical procedure; therefore, as for all surgical procedures, its successful completion requires a thorough knowledge of anatomy (Fig. 1.1).

Before inserting a laparoscope, the experienced gynecologist should know

– The gross anatomy of the pelvic organs, which are "caught by surprise," so to speak, in their normal physiologic position

– The anatomical landmarks of the internal genitalia and other pelvic structures lying in close proximity to the ureters, the iliac vessels, etc.

– Pathological anatomy—that is, the visual recognition of diseased organs or pathological conditions

Anterior abdominal wall

Descriptive anatomy

Stretching from the thoracic cage to the pelvic girdle, the anterior abdominal wall is a soft, contractile, compliant tissue consisting of skin, subcutaneous tissues, muscles and fascia, the fascia transversalis thickening toward the pubis, and the peritoneum.

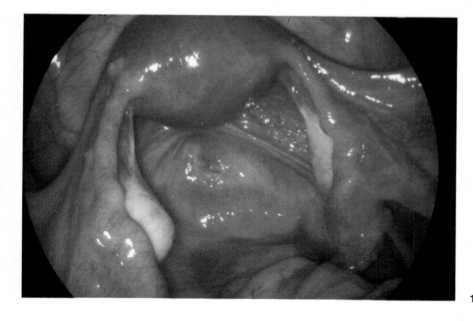

1.1 Panoramic view of a normal pelvis.

Three anatomical structures are worth considering:

Linea alba

The linea alba is a median raphe formed by the medial aspect of the rectus muscles and by the decussations of the fibers from the fascia. It extends from the xyphoid to the pubic symphysis and is wider in its upper half, particularly at the umbilicus, where the peritoneum adheres to it.

Inferior epigastric vessels

The inferior epigastric arteries arise from the medial side of the external iliac arteries, a few millimeters above the inguinal ligament. In general, their paths follow a line drawn between the midpoint of the inguinal ligaments and the umbilicus. They first run medially, then arch in a cephalad and medial direction toward the umbilicus. The round ligament crosses the convex side of these arches before entering the inguinal canal. The inferior epigastric vessels reach the lateral border of the rectus muscles about 5 cm above the pubis. They then penetrate the fascia of the rectus muscle up to the umbilicus, where they disperse within the muscle. They are always lateral to the umbilicial arteries.

Urinary bladder

The adult urinary bladder is a strictly retropubic organ when empty. Indeed, it is demarcated anteriorly by the prevesical space of Retzius, the pubic symphysis and pubic bones, the anterior part of the levator ani muscle, the aponeurosis of these muscles and their blood vessels.

Practical implications

The main insufflation sites are as follows:
- *The right and left iliac fossae*, which should be avoided because of the risk of lacerating the inferior epigastric vessels.
- *The suprapubic area*, which we never use so as not to risk trauma to the bladder.
- *The mid-hypogastric area*, which should also be avoided because there the loosely adherent peritoneum can contribute to a subfascial insufflation.
- *The left epigastric area*, about 3 cm lateral to the navel and 2 cm inferior to the left costal margin, may be an attractive site in cases of previous midline subumbilical laparotomy scar—but it is contraindicated in case of splenomegaly (rare, yet worthy of consideration).
- *The intraumbilical site* is preferred because the peritoneum adheres to the aponeurotic tissues of the linea alba there and the risk of subfascial preperitoneal insufflation is consequently minimal.
- *Others*: cul-de-sac, transuterine.

Laparoscopy

In order to reduce the risk of postoperative umbilical herniation, it is best to follow a "Z" track when inserting the umbilical trocar and sleeve.

Selection of secondary lower puncture sites (Fig. 1.2)

These puncture sites must be placed within a triangular space demarcated by
- The dome of the bladder (base of triangle)
- The two umbilical arteries (sides of triangle)

This avascular zone is optimal for just about all laparoscopic procedures; injury to any of the epigastric vessels can thereby be confidently prevented; a careful secondary puncture technique performed under direct laparoscopic vision within the triangle is particularly important whenever a patient has had multiple previous laparotomies or has an enlarged uterus. It may also be preferable, in those cases, to place these second-puncture trocars a bit higher in order to facilitate and maintain easy access to the cul-de-sac.

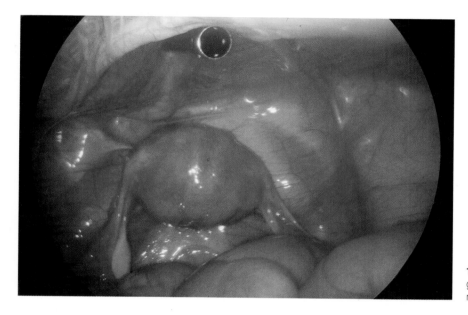

1.2 A trocar is introduced in the "security triangle," which is delineated by the two umbilical ligaments and the dome of the bladder.

Posterior abdominal wall

Descriptive anatomy

The posterior abdominal wall encompasses mainly the bony structures of the spine and the large vessels, the aorta and vena cava inferior with their bifurcation. Within the abdominal cavity, the anatomic relationships are variable, because the intra-abdominal organs are mobile within the cavity. In addition, the abdominal cavity is, in physiologic terms, a "space" rather than a true cavity. There are two important notions to remember with regard to laparoscopy: first, the aorta is closer to the anterior abdominal wall than to the operating table and, second, the location of the umbilicus with regard to the promontorium and the aortic bifurcation is variable, depending on the degree of flexion of the pelvis and the distance between pubis and umbilicus.

Practical implications

Bowel lesions cannot be prevented by elevation of the abdominal wall because there is no true cavity; therefore bowel loops will follow any curvature imposed on the abdominal wall. However, elevation of the anterior abdominal wall does increase the distance between the tip of the Verres needle and the large retroperitoneal vessels. This is of benefit, especially when the patient is thin or when she has a flaccid abdominal wall.

Pelvic side walls

Descriptive anatomy

Endosurgical procedures in the pelvis most commonly involve the ovary and tube. The structures of the pelvic side wall have a well-defined relationship with the adnexa.

Iliac vessels

We describe further how the iliac vessels partly delineate the ovarian fossa. In the nulliparous woman, the distal end of the tube is located only about 1 cm beneath the level of the iliac vessels. This distance increases with parity.

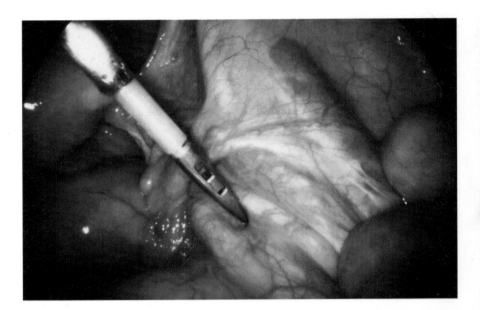

1.3 Right ureter at the level of the pelvic brim.

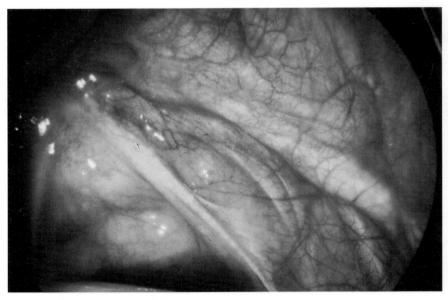

1.4 Right ureter above the microuterine ligament. The ureter is a landmark for the ovarian and infra-ovarian fossa.

Ureters (Figs. 1.3 and 1.4)

The ureter has a direct relationship to the ovary in the following ways (Figs. 1.5 and 1.6):

— In the nulliparous patient, the lateral aspect of the ovary corresponds to the ovarian fossa, which is surrounded by the hypogastric vessels and ureter, which form the posterior border; the cardinal ligament, which is located in front of the fossa; the external iliac vessels, which delineate the lateral margin; and the obliterated umbilical and uterine arteries, which run below. Beneath the peritoneum at the base of the ovarian fossa stretches the obturator lymphatic chain.

— In the multiparous patient, the lateral aspect of the ovary corresponds to the infraovarian fossa, which is surrounded by the ureter and uterine artery in the front and the edge of the sacrum in the back. The sacrouterine ligament forms the lower limit.

The ureter also has a definite relationship to the distal portion of the oviduct. The ampulla tubae crosses the cranial pole of the ovary at the level of the ureter, and the infundibulum can often be seen overlying the ureter.

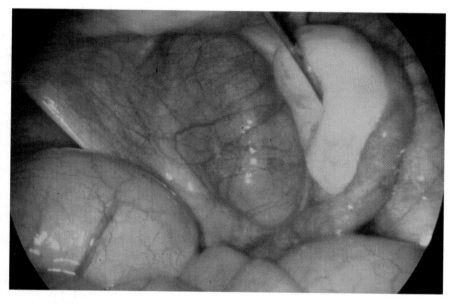

1.5 Ovarian fossa in a nulliparous woman.

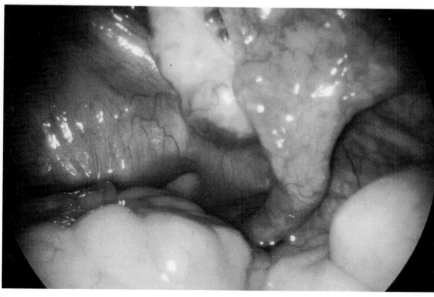

1.6 Normal anatomic relation of fallopian tube, ovary, and cul-de-sac.

Practical implications

The parietal peritoneum, at the level of the ovarian fossa or thereabouts, is often involved in pathologic conditions such as endometriosis and adhesions. These pathologic conditions alter the peritoneum, which becomes opaque. They also sometimes alter the anatomic relationship of the retroperitoneal structures. Therefore surgery must be performed cautiously. The course of the ureter and the iliac vessels, which is sometimes difficult to assess, should be kept in mind at all times. When electrosurgery is used, bipolar instruments are preferred over monopolar ones, because the thermal spread of the latter is more pronounced. Adhesiolysis between the lateral aspect of the ovary and the pelvic side wall can be difficult. Sometimes the ovarian cortex is incised or, worse, the peritoneum is opened and the region of the iliac bifurcation is then entered. Further intervention should be avoided at that point.

In our experience, injury of the infundibulopelvic ligament is an infrequent but not rare event, because the distal end of the fallopian tube and the infundibulopelvic ligament lie close together. This anatomic relationship is even more evident when there are adhesions between the oviduct and the lateral pelvic wall above the level of the cranial pole of the ovary.

A clear picture of these anatomic relationships must always be kept in mind during surgery. Sometimes, during a difficult adhesiolysis, it is difficult to find the anatomic landmarks, especially on the left side. Therefore, to avoid accidents, it is advisable to zoom out frequently in order to obtain a panoramic view of the field. Thorough rinsing of the site also increases the likelihood of good orientation. Adhesiolysis can then be continued under optimal conditions.

Cul-de-sac (pouch of Douglas) (Fig. 1.6)

The posterior wall of the upper portion of the vagina corresponds to the abdominal cul-de-sac. The peritoneum covers the vaginal wall over a distance of approximately 15 mm. The distance between the vagina and the abdominal cavity is minimal, on the order of 4 mm. The posterior fornix is therefore an excellent place in which to establish a pneumoperitoneum in obese patients. However, use of this access is contraindicated if adhesions are likely to be present, especially if endometriosis is suspected.

Conclusion

Although a thorough knowledge of anatomy is, in our opinion, mandatory, we would like to put the surgical risk into perspective. We have not yet caused any lesion of the external iliac vessels or the ureter. Knowledge of the topographic anatomy should not deter but rather enhance the performance of endosurgical procedures.

2
Prerequisites
for laparoscopic surgery

As we indicated previously, we believe that operative laparoscopy is a surgical procedure presenting requirements similar to those of laparotomy:
- The operating theater must be either a standard operating room or an endoscopy suite large enough for laparotomy procedures.
- OR personnel must be qualified and properly trained.
- Instrumentation must be appropriate, up to date, and meticulously maintained.

Patient safety depends not only on the skills of the surgeon but also on the quality of the operating environment. The room must be adequately staffed and supplied. Laparoscopy has no place in a "minor procedure" room. The nursing staff must be dedicated to laparoscopic surgery and familiar with the instruments. High-quality anesthesia (see Chapter 5) must be available.

Contraindications to laparoscopic surgery

Absolute contraindications are as follows:
- A pelvic mass rising above the umbilicus
- Prior laparotomy for intestinal fistula, complex urological procedures, major oncologic procedures followed by radiotherapy, extensive peritoneal tuberculosis

Relative contraindications include
- Prior laparotomy, which requires strict precautions (see Chapter 3) to avoid intestinal injury. Obesity is more a technical difficulty than a contraindication.
- Difficult insufflation (i.e., an insufflation pressure greater than 20 mmHg).
- Anesthetic contraindications, which are more common and are discussed in Chapter 5.

The indications and contraindications for various laparoscopic operations are reviewed in the pertinent chapters.

Laparoscopic equipment

Insufflators

A good pneumoperitoneum guarantees good viewing of the pelvic organs, but excessive intra-abdominal pressure is a major hazard in laparoscopy and the cause of severe complications. To avoid such problems, one must have an insufflator built according to modern safety standards.

Two types of insufflators are available: traditional semiautomatic and newer, electronic machines.

Semiautomatic insufflators

A traditional semiautomatic insufflator is composed of the following parts:

— A *manometer*, which measures the insufflation pressure or the intra-abdominal pressure. Measuring the intra-abdominal pressure is more useful but requires a secondary channel during insufflation. Under ordinary circumstances, the manometer reads the insufflation pressure during insufflation and the intra-abdominal pressure when insufflation is stopped.

— A *flowmeter*, which measures the volume of insufflation—a figure that is proportional to the difference between the insufflation pressure and the intra-abdominal pressure.

— A *manual insufflation setting*, meaning that a set volume, independent of the resistance to the flow, can be insufflated. We will see later that use of this setting at the beginning of laparoscopy is critical to verifying proper positioning of the Verres needle.

— An *automatic insufflation setting*, used throughout the remainder of the laparoscopy, that can provide and maintain a specific intra-abdominal pressure (e.g., 15 mmHg) determined by the operator. Response of this pressure-dependent mechanism is relatively slow, and the maximum flow rate is insufficient to compensate for rapid loss of large volumes of gas such as occur, for example, during rinsing and aspiration of debris.

— A *rapid insufflation setting*, which is controlled manually and is capable of pumping a large volume of gas into the abdominal cavity against relatively high resistance. This setting should be maintained for only 20 to 30 s at a time, with measurements of intra-abdominal pressure being performed at these intervals.

— A *pressure gauge*, which indicates the level of gas in the gas tank and lessens the risk of running out of gas during laparoscopic intervention.

Electronic insufflators (Fig. 2.1)

These instruments maintain a preset intra-abdominal pressure by varying the insufflation rate. To avoid the necessity of two channels—one for insufflation and one for measurement—the insufflation is performed in a series of intermittent "bursts." The volume insufflated is then determined by three variables: (1) the intra-abdominal pressure measured by the apparatus, (2) the maximum insufflation rate permitted, and (3) the preset intra-abdominal pressure that has been determined by the operator.

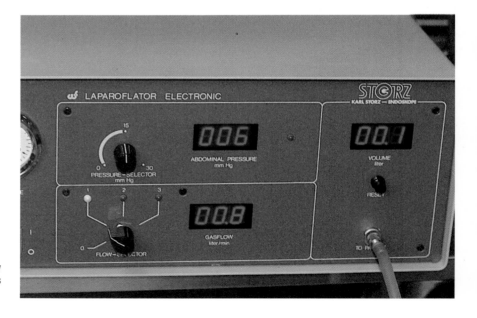

2.1 Pressure readings on the insufflator: the flow (0.8 L/min) is high and the pressure (6 mmHg) is low. The needle is in the peritoneal cavity.

Electronic insufflators are ideal for operative endoscopy and have two main advantages: (1) they ensure a constant monitoring of pressures, an important safety factor, and (2) they are able to compensate, instantaneously and without excessive pressure, for leaks up to 6 liters per minute. Even in the "high-flow" mode, intra-abdominal pressure is constantly monitored, a particular advantage during irrigation/aspiration or evacuation of the smoke produced (e.g., by the CO_2 laser). A disadvantage is that at the beginning of insufflation close contact between the Verres needle and the bowel or omentum may cause a falsely elevated intra-abdominal pressure reading, resulting in arrest of insufflation. Gentle repositioning of the needle or elevation of the abdominal wall will alleviate this difficulty—a problem that no longer occurs once 200 to 300 mL of gas has been instilled. When the needle is not placed correctly, insufflation will not occur, thus avoiding retroperitoneal emphysema. This, however, should not preclude the performance of regular safety checks.

The actual volume of gas insufflated is of little importance. Intra-abdominal capacity is influenced by many variables: the weight, height, and build of the patient; the drugs used for anesthesia; and, above all, the presence or absence of leaks.

In conclusion, safety requirements call for the use of semiautomatic or automatic insufflators, which make possible the constant monitoring of insufflation or intra-abdominal pressure. Pioneer instruments having constant-flow insufflation are obsolete. For operative procedures, the automatic, electronic instruments are most appropriate because they are handy and safe.

Optics

Without an adequate view of the pelvis, endosurgery is impossible. The so-called panoramic (i.e., wide-angle) field of view is preferable. A 0° optic is necessary. An optic with an angled field of view produces an asymmetric angle of rotation, which complicates the manipulation of the suprapubic instruments. Surgery is already hindered by absence of depth perception with a monocular optic and by a focal length setting at infinity.

Single-puncture laparoscopy with an operative channel should be replaced by the use of suprapubic trocars.

Surgical instruments (Figs. 2.2 and 2.3)

Laparoscopic surgery requires certain unique surgical manipulations that demand specially designed instrumentation. The tools for endoscopic surgery are numerous and often complex. They are very specific to their purpose and demand conscientious care and maintenance. A complete set of instruments includes a variety of forceps and scissors as well as others which we shall describe.

Atraumatic grasping forceps

The shape of their tips closely resembles that of the graspers used in conventional surgery, with five essential characteristics:
- A fine tip, permitting precise application
- Atraumatic but not smooth jaws

– Operating mechanism that permits them to be used for blunt dissection by opening the jaws

– A mechanism (ratchet) permitting a steady, stable grasp that can be easily released

– Capability of being connected to an electrosurgical unit

A set of graspers with jaws of different lengths is indispensable; the long jaws are useful for blunt dissection and for prolonged holding of tissues atraumatically; the short jaws are better adapted for precise fine-tissue handling and electrocoagulation.

Toothed grasping forceps

These permit effective grasp of nonfragile organs and structures, such as the ovaries or leiomyomata. They are very useful when, for example, the ovary must be stabilized. Different types of toothed forceps may be used, according to the degree of grasping force required. Fine-toothed forceps cause very little trauma and are used on a daily basis in our department.

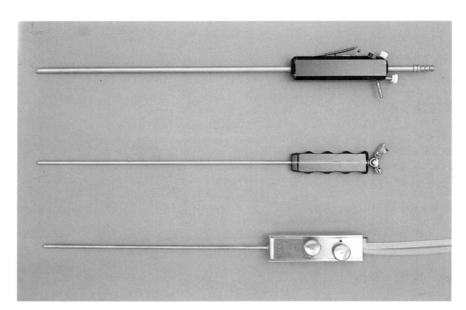

2.2 Suction-irrigation probes (*top* to *bottom*): the Triton, the small Triton, and aquapurator.

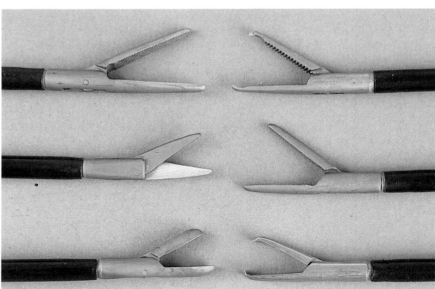

2.3 Instrumentation. Left series (*top* to *bottom*): atraumatic grasping forceps (long jaws), scissors, and biopsy forceps. Right series (*top* to *bottom*): toothed grasping forceps, atraumatic grasping forceps (short jaws), and claw forceps ("grip-pince" in French).

Scissors

Scissors should be capable, as in conventional surgery, of both cutting and blunt dissection. Their points should be similar to those of scissors of the Metzenbaum type. The blades must be at least 12 mm long, to allow for sufficiently wide, active separation. Rounded, sharp-edged scissors must be used with care, because their hooklike extremity can cause inadvertent damage to vital structures.

Palpation probe

This instrument is unknown in traditional surgery. It is of only limited interest in endoscopic surgery (e.g., in cases of pelvic inflammatory disease). Even then, we would prefer to use atraumatic forceps instead. A probe should be at least 5 mm in diameter.

Suction-irrigation apparatus

This is truly a unique and indispensable tool in endosurgery for evacuating blood clots and pus and for washing the pelvis in order to provide a cleaner, more easily visible operative field. Prerequisites for good suction-irrigation apparatus are

- Combination of suction and irrigation mechanisms in a single tool
- Easy switching from suction to irrigation and vice versa
- Irrigation under high pressure
- Powerful suction via a channel of large diameter

The Triton is a tool that meets all these requirements. It allows irrigation with saline solution under variable pressures of 1 to 2 bars and permits suctioning through a channel 6 mm in diameter. It also has a retractable electrocoagulation needle. All functions are controlled by the operator's hand or foot. A simplified version, 5 mm in diameter (Petit Triton), allows suction and irrigation only. A more complex prototype (the Poltron) is being developed by the Synergy Company (Vichy 03, France).

Methods of hemostasis

Hemostasis has always been a major problem in endoscopic surgery. Following below are available techniques.

Monopolar surgery

Electrosurgery permits bloodless incisions and hemostasis by coagulation, either mono- or bipolar. *Monopolar electrosurgery* was introduced in laparoscopy quite early in its development, but a relatively high number of complications have discredited this cost-effective and efficient mode of energy. If used for coagulation, the following rules must be observed:

- The tip of the forceps must be fine, to allow precise application of the current.
- Coagulation must be performed only under good visual control.
- Coagulation in the vicinity of vital structures (such as ureter or bowel) is absolutely prohibited.
- The operator should use the lowest power setting that is effective.
- The apparatus should be shut down and the instrument removed when not in use. Most incidents occur through inadvertent activation of the foot pedal.

Monopolar cutting obviously requires identical precautions, with the addition of the following:

– The electrodes should be fine, for precise and rapid cutting.

– The electrodes should be retractable within a protective sheath, for increased safety.

– Section should be performed by brushing against rather than pushing into the tissue.

Bipolar electrocoagulation

Bipolar electrosurgery almost completely eliminates the risk of inadvertent burns. Unfortunately, the instruments currently available are awkward and bulky, making them less than suitable for fine microsurgical-type tubal surgery. We recently developed a bipolar forceps that is almost identical to microsurgical tweezers, permitting fine hemostasis.

Electrocautery

Electrocautery with the outmoded diathermy loop should no longer be used.

Thermocoagulation

This technique was developed initially by Semm. Tissues are coagulated by direct application of heat through an instrument that is electrically insulated. Several instruments have been designed (e.g., a crocodile forceps, a point coagulator). These instruments are used either to obtain hemostasis prior to dissection (for example, salpingectomy or salpingostomy) or to destroy tissue such as endometriotic nodules.

Endoscopic ligatures

Semm's endoloop and endoligature permit ligation of large vessels or large pedicles. It is a relatively complex technique that we do not utilize.

Chemical hemostasis

This is performed using ornithine-8-vasopressin (Por 8, Sandoz, Basel, Switzerland), 5 units per 20 to 40 mL of saline. Vasoconstriction is obtained for about 2 h when the material is carefully infiltrated into the extravascular space. This permits the natural mechanism of coagulation to occur. Inadvertent intravascular injection can lead to severe complications such as hypertensive crisis or cardiac arrhythmias, which are difficult to correct. Rarely, even an extravascular injection may trigger a mild to moderate increase in blood pressure and transient bradycardia.

Chemical hemostasis complements other methods of hemostasis well.

CO_2 laser

Use of the CO_2 laser was recently introduced in laparoscopy, permitting section with concurrent coagulation of small vessels. Tissue such as endometriotic implants can be vaporized and superficial coagulation of larger areas performed. This is discussed in Chapter 11.

Specificity of laparoscopic apparatus and instruments

The instruments used for laparoscopic surgery have characteristics quite different from those of instruments used for conventional surgery.

Electrical insulation of laparoscopic instruments

This is a precaution necessary to ensure patients' safety.

Multifunctional instruments

Rapid exchange of instruments is an integral part of conventional surgery. The technician hands the instruments to the surgeon, ideally without being asked to do so. In endosurgery, this was made possible by the advent of video monitoring and also by the development of multifunctional instruments such as the Triton (suction, rinsing, coagulation, section, manipulation) or the laser (section, coagulation, and vaporization). Although initially somewhat cumbersome for the operator, their saving of time and increased safety earn these instruments a quick welcome.

Standardized trocar size

Instruments must be passed through trocars of a fixed inner diameter. In order to avoid changing trocars—an awkward and annoying task—it is advisable to use instruments of the same diameter, usually 5 mm. Some instruments, however, cannot be reduced in size (e.g., the Triton and the Yoon band applicator, both of which require a trocar having an inner diameter of 7 mm).

Length of instruments

The length of ancillary instruments is the result of a compromise: if too long, they are cumbersome and awkward to handle; if too short, they are difficult to maneuver precisely.

3

Initial maneuvers

This chapter deals with the initial steps of all laparoscopic interventions. Details pertaining to a particular indication are dealt with, when appropriate, in Chapters 8–17.

Positioning the patient (Figs. 3.1 and 3.2)

Positioning is important to permit optimal mobility of the ancillary instruments and thus optimal outcome of the surgery. The classic lithotomy position, with flexed thighs, is to be avoided, because it prevents proper use of the suprapubic trocars. We recommend the following position:

– Flat lithotomy position, legs abducted and stretched.
– Buttocks at the edge of the table to allow easy manipulation of the uterus and access to the rectum.
– Shoulder brace in place.
– Arm on the operator's side fixed alongside the patient's body.
– No partition between anesthetist and surgeon. Once intubated, the patient's head is turned away from the operator, to the opposite side. The patient's head can be protected by use of a low, solid hoop.

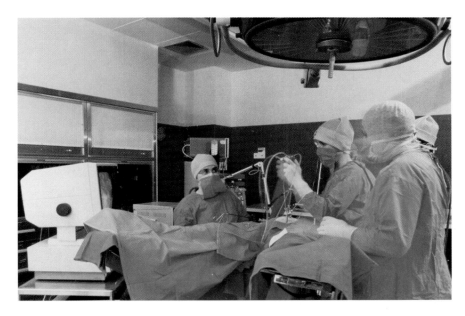

3.1 Positioning of the patient. The patient lies flat, in modified lithotomy and slight Trendelenburg. The surgeon operates off the screen.

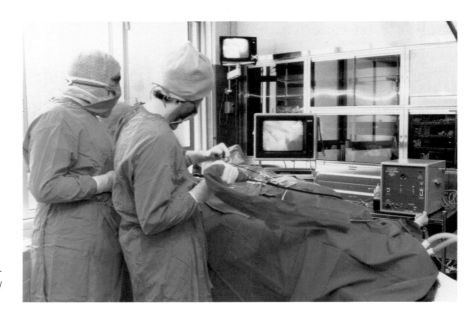

3.2 Positioning of the patient. Note the Trendelenburg position. Both the operator and assistant stay on the patient's left side.

This positioning permits proper insertion of suprapubic trocars and instruments, which is of utmost importance for successful endosurgery. An assistant helps the surgeon, much as during laparotomy. Current video techniques allow the assistant to anticipate surgical moves, rather than performing them blindly on request.

Manipulation of the uterus (Fig. 3.3)

Manipulation of the uterus can be performed either by inserting a Hegar dilator (or curette), which is then taped to a tenaculum, or by installing a suction cannula, which also permits chromopertubation of the oviducts. Intrauterine manipulation is contraindicated in the presence of an intrauterine pregnancy and, to a lesser degree, in patients at risk for developing pelvic inflammatory disease (PID).

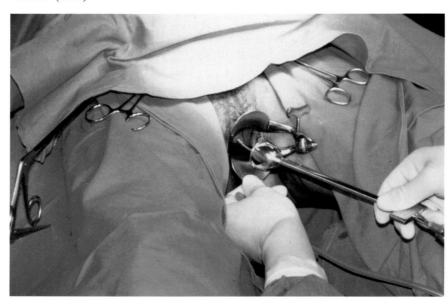

3.3 A cannula is placed into the uterine cavity and fixed onto the cervix by vacuum. A pertubation of the tubes can be performed through this cannula.

Trendelenburg position

This position is routinely utilized. An angle between 10° and 15° is adequate for the majority of cases. A steeper Trendelenburg is seldom or only intermittently required.

One can equate the pneumoperitoneum and Trendelenburg position with the retractors and towels of laparotomy. Without retraction (i.e., good exposure), there is no laparoscopic surgery.

Trendelenburg positioning should be initiated at the time the laparoscope is introduced.

Insufflation

Insufflation is carried out with the Verres needle and requires particular attention so as to avoid complications.

Checking the needle

The operator verifies that the spring mechanism is not hampered and that the needle is freely patent and sharp.

Site of insertion (Figs. 3.4 and 3.5)

Advantages and risks of the different sites of insertion are discussed in Chapter 1.

The intraumbilical site is preferable in most cases. Insertion within the left iliac fossa exposes the external iliac vessels to risk of injury and should not be used. Access through the cul-de-sac is handy in obese patients but is contraindicated when pelvic adhesions are anticipated, especially when endometriosis is suspected. In the presence of previous abdominal surgery, we opt for the umbilical route when the scar is of the Pfannenstiel type and for the left hypochondrium if the scar is of the low-median type.

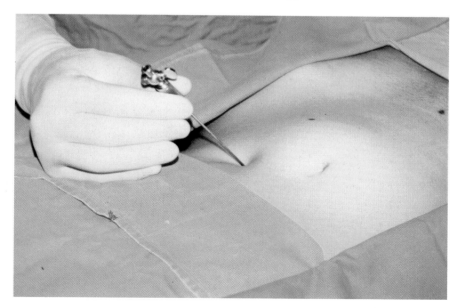

3.4 The four sites of insufflation on the abdominal wall: we use only the umbilical or left lateral sites. The latter access is chosen in case of previous midline incision.

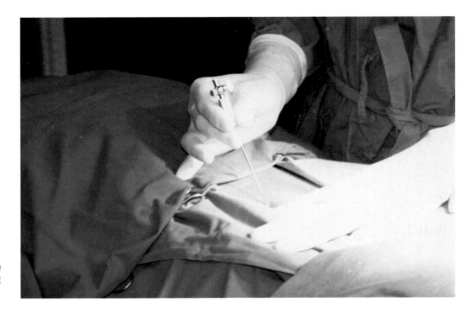

3.5 Insertion of the Palmer (Verres) needle through the umbilicus. The surgeon is careful not to hamper the action of the spring mechanism.

Method of insertion (Figs. 3.4 through 3.8)

The needle is introduced slowly at an angle of approximately 45°. The needle is held so as to avoid blocking the spring mechanism. At the level of the umbilicus, the operator should note the piercing of two anatomic layers. This number increases to three at the level of the left hypochondrium. Elevating the abdominal wall does not increase the distance between the bowel and peritoneum because the celomic cavity is not a true cavity. However, elevating the abdominal wall does decrease the risk of injury to the large vessels. The needle is then held at 90° rather than 45°. We choose this method only when the patient is tiny or has a flabby abdominal wall (e.g., postpartum). Once the needle is introduced, manipulation is avoided until visualization can be achieved with the endoscope.

Checking the position of the needle

Several tests are designed to determine the position of the needle prior to, during, or after creation of the pneumoperitoneum.

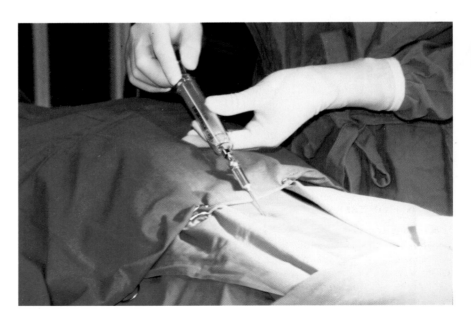

3.6 Syringe test. This is performed regardless of the operator's level of experience. Aspiration (as demonstrated) does not yield gas or fluid when the needle is properly placed into the peritoneal cavity.

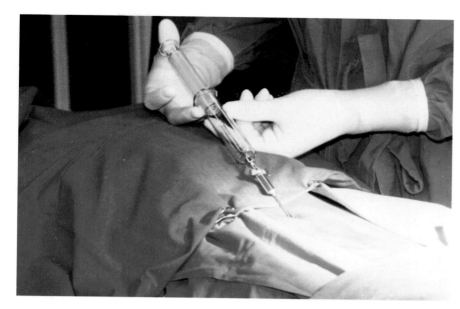

3.7 Twenty milliliters of air are injected under pressure. Reaspiration should not be possible because the gas readily diffuses into the large abdominal cavity.

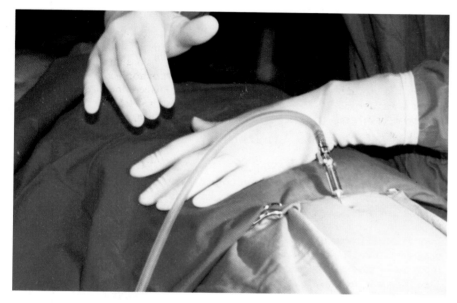

3.8 Percussion at the level of the liver quickly (20 to 30 s) yields tympanism.

Prior to insufflation

The syringe test is composed of three steps:
  − Suction should yield no liquid (bowel content, blood) or gas.
  − Injection of ± 20 mL physiologic solution is performed without noticeable resistance.
  − Repeat suction should not reaspirate the injected fluid, because it should have spread within the abdominal cavity.

During insufflation

With a semiautomatic insufflator

Continuous monitoring of the insufflation pressure is mandatory. This is feasible only in the "manual" position, when insufflation is not suppressed by the intra-abdominal pressure. The flow should be high (>1 L) and the pressure low ($\leqslant 15$ to 20 mmHg). Excessive pressure calls for removal of the needle and reinsertion. Brisk variations in pressure readings indicate that the needle may be caught in the omentum or is placed retroperitoneally. Percussion of the abdomen and disappearance of the hepatic dullness (in ± 20 s) are the best indicator of a good distribution of the gas throughout the abdominal cavity.

With an automatic insufflator

The initial pressure reading should be less than 12 mmHg. When the needle is malpositioned, insufflation stops and the pressure reading exceeds 20 mmHg.

After insufflation

The position of the Verres needle should be checked as soon as the endoscope is in place. Even when all rules for insertion of the needle have been observed, retroperitoneal insufflation can occur. If the endoscope has been successfully placed within the abdominal cavity, insufflation should be continued through the trocar and the extraperitoneal gas evacuated through a suprapubic trocar. If the endoscope did not reach the abdominal cavity, the emphysema should be evacuated through the trocar first, the Verres needle introduced at a different site and, after successful insufflation, the trocar reinserted.

Establishment of the pneumoperitoneum in case of previous laparotomy

Our technique is based on two principles. First, we believe that incidental injury of the bowel with a needle is without consequence and should not be repaired. Second, the main potential risk for bowel injury is linked to the insertion of the trocar. Insufflation is performed through the umbilicus or at the level of the left hypochondrium (lower midline scar), as previously described. Insertion of the first-puncture trocar is preceded by the needle test. A 20-mL syringe, half filled with physiologic solution, is fitted to an 18- to 22-gauge needle. At regular intervals around the umbilicus, the operator inserts the needle completely and then slowly withdraws it, at the same time aspirating slightly with the syringe. At a certain consistent depth, CO_2 gas should be obtained at all test sites. If an adhesion is present beneath a particular test area around the umbilicus, either no gas at all will be aspirated or gas aspiration will occur at a level deeper than that of other test sites. This needle test is used to explore a triangular area ($5 \times 5 \times 5$ cm) around and below the umbilicus.

Open laparoscopy provides no additional safeguards to the technique described above. Every surgeon has experienced the case where minimal bowel lesions occur at laparotomy, when extensive parietal adhesions must be dissected, and this despite maximum exposure through a large skin incision. Using the test described above, laparoscopy was judged to be technically impossible in 10 out of 1000 cases with previous laparotomies; in the remaining 990 cases, no bowel perforation occurred. A point in favor of open laparoscopy is that bowel injury is readily recognized, whereas for all other methods, piercing of the bowel can go unnoticed. Whenever the needle test fails to reveal a periumbilical zone free of parietal adhesions, we believe that laparoscopy should not be performed and that every case should be reevaluated for the necessity of exploratory laparotomy. When areas of positive testing alternate with zones of negative testing, the trocar should be introduced in a zone presumed to be free of adhesions.

In conclusion, insufflation remains a blind procedure. Safety checks are mandatory, and their result is either positive or negative; there is no gray zone. If in doubt, consider the test to be positive and refrain from introducing the trocar in that particular area.

Insertion of the first-puncture trocar (Fig. 3.9)

The first-puncture trocar is inserted through either the inferior or left lateral border of the umbilicus. The "bayonet," or "Z" type, insertion is preferred over straight insertion. In the former, defects in the skin and fascia are not directly aligned one above the other, and thus there is less risk of umbilical hernia.

Most importantly, one should avoid brisk and deep insertion. This is done by
– Stretching the index finger along the trocar sleeve or holding the trocar with both hands.
– Rotating the trocar while inserting it through the abdomen. This reduces the amount of force applied.
– Using sharp instruments, which lessen the force needed to pierce the integument and structures of the anterior abdominal wall.

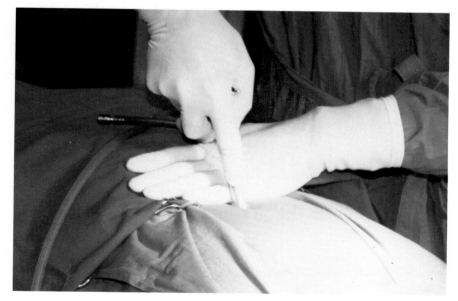

3.9 Insertion of the first-puncture trocar. To control the depth of penetration, a slight rotating motion is added to the forward movement.

Insertion of the second-puncture trocars (Fig. 3.10)

Suprapubic sites of access are the cornerstones of accurate visualization and precise surgery. Most commonly used instruments are 5 or 7 mm in diameter.

Some trocars are fitted with a screwlike thread on the outer sheath, which increases their stability.

Trocars without a valve (or with a piston valve) present the advantage that, if desired, a drain can be inserted at the end of the procedure.

Insertion of the second-puncture trocars must be done under direct visualization, medially from the epigastric vessels or, even better, within the "triangle of safety" (see Chapter 1). Two simple rules   be observed:

– Insertion is performed 1 to 3 cm above the theoretical Pfannenstiel incision. One should take into account the volume of the uterus, which, when enlarged, can hamper access to the cul-de-sac if the suprapubic puncture sites are too low.

– The minimal distance between two suprapubic trocars is 5 to 6 cm. At shorter distances, instruments would hinder one another.

The length of the skin incision should not exceed the diameter of the trocar, so that the friction with the surrounding skin makes it fit snugly and prevents slipping of the trocar too far inside the abdomen. A trocar that constantly slips over the end of ancillary instruments hinders their manipulation. Screwlike threads add to the stability of the trocar.

The right suprapubic trocar is generally introduced first. In fact, the left adnexa is often hidden by the rectocolon, which is best manipulated when accessed from the right lateral side. Before surgery is initiated, a left lateral suprapubic trocar should be inserted.

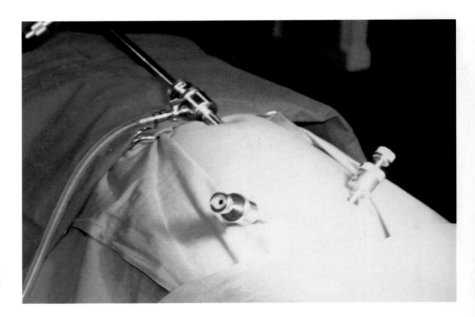

3.10 Second-puncture trocars are introduced in the suprapubic region. The distance between them is approximately 7 to 10 cm.

Exploration of the peritoneal cavity

Exploration is systematically performed, including the upper abdomen. For atraumatic manipulation of the pelvic and abdominal organs, we use a grasping forceps with long blades.

4

Video monitoring
and laparoscopy

Physicians have spent considerable time in documenting operative procedures, using different modalities. Classically dictated operative reports are obviously subject to the operator's biased interpretation. Visual documentation, such as video or photography, is an objective method of documentation. Monitors in the operating room permit surgeons to operate while their movements are monitored on the screen rather than through the laparoscope. This is the beginning of a new era of surgical *video endoscopy*.

Technological breakthroughs of recent years have given the physician several new options for visual documentation. However, one must distinguish the practical, easily applicable innovations from the complex, sophisticated equipment whose usefulness still remains to be proved.

The purpose of this chapter is to help the reader understand the usefulness of the great variety of equipment available.

Advantages of video endoscopy

A new technique is interesting only if it brings an advantage to the patient and her physician. Although video monitoring brings no apparent and obvious advantage to the surgery as such, there are other aspects to consider, especially in the evaluation and follow-up of disease processes.

Advantages of this new type of documentation

The objectivity of the data as recorded on video represents the main advantage, even if the operator expresses a certain bias—as, for example, by selecting a certain passage. Nonetheless, the image seen is real at that particular time. Documentation is no longer subject to the recollection of the surgeon or the memory of an assistant.

This objectivity in gathering data promotes the following:
- Open discussion of procedures with colleagues
- Education of residents
- Self-education of the surgeon
- New type of medical file on optical disks and PC
- New patient-physician relationship

Advantages of the technique

Surgery utilizing video monitoring to guide the operator's movements increases the surgeon's comfort by reducing the strain on his or her back. This is all the more appreciated, in view of the fact that newer developments have tended to increase operating time. Improved resolution of the video cameras allows detailed inspection of the anatomic structures. Magnification is possible with added lenses and brings a microsurgical dimension to the methodology.

More importantly, video screens have brought the concept of teamwork back into the operating theater. The assistant assumes a more active role, instead of passively and blindly executing orders. The anesthesiologist becomes involved and more readily accepts operating times and patient positions that previously seemed inadvisable. The scrub technician can follow the intervention and anticipate moves. The care of instruments improves because of a better understanding of their function. Finally, continuous use of the video system permits documentation at any given time.

Disadvantages of video endoscopy

The use of video techniques in endoscopy brings certain disadvantages:
- First of all, such systems are still quite expensive. The increase in the number and variety of systems now available has lowered the cost somewhat, but at the expense of making the choice of a system more difficult.
- Maintenance of video equipment is a considerable problem, both financially and technically. It is assumed that both nurses and physicians are instructed in the correct use of the equipment.
- The video screen adds yet another element to the already complex setup of an endoscopy suite and presents still another challenge to the physician in mastering spatial coordination.

Methods and materials

Equipment

The use of video monitoring should inspire the physician to learn some basic facts of optics and electronics. Video endoscopy involves more than a camera. One must consider every element included in the system: light source, camera, light cable, endoscope, monitor, recorder, etc. Each element contributes to the quality of the final product—the recorded image.

The determining factor in visual documentation is the intensity of light available at any point in the system:
- Wattage of the light source
- Efficiency of the light transport (endoscope and cable)
- Sensitivity of the camera
- Size of the template for recording

Light source

The intensity of currently available light sources is sufficient to generate an electronic image of good quality. Two different types of light source are available:

— Sources using incandescent light (4500 K) result in images with near-real color, but their intensity is often limited; 250 W is the required power for video endoscopy.

— Electric arc light sources (6000 K) result in images with a blue overtone but provide higher intensities.

The introduction of cameras in endoscopy required the development of light sources of increasingly high intensities. Some of these light sources quickly produce a great deal of heat— $\geq 120°C$ at the tip of the endoscope! It is therefore imperative, before purchasing a particular light source, that the temperature at the tip of the endoscope be checked after several minutes of use.

The light intensity of these sources is usually insufficient for photography, which requires a flash. Many manufacturers offer sources with integrated, electronically modulated flash. Such a flash generates a peak intensity in accordance with information received from the still photography camera. During endoscopic interventions, the object-lens distance varies constantly and, with it, the light intensity required. A panoramic view of the pelvis requires a large amount of light, whereas closeup views require very little. Some light sources are equipped with a device that receives light information from the camera, automatically adjusting light intensity to the requirements of any particular view. This is called an *automatic intensity regulator*. It is an extremely convenient feature, especially when working frequently at close distance.

We would recommend the use of a xenon light source equipped with an automatic intensity regulator and a flash generator.

Method of transmission

Transmission encompasses the endoscope and light cables. The light is carried toward the object and the image transmitted back to the recording system. Light energy is lost at every connection along the way. The sum of all losses determines the efficiency of the system. There are two types of light cable: *fiberoptic* and *fluid*. The latter contains a gel (instead of fibers) that transmits the light. We prefer the fluid light cables because they are sturdier as well as more efficient. An endoscope is made up of a series of thin lenses. The smaller these lenses are, the less light they will transmit. It is therefore advisable to use endoscopes of at least 10 mm in diameter.

Camera

Video cameras currently available are of three different types:
— Tube camera
— CCD (charge-coupled device) camera
— MOS and nMOS (meta-oxide semiconduction and negative MOS) camera

The tube camera is extremely sensitive but has a relatively low resolution. The image's color is realistic. Because these cameras are relatively large and cumbersome, they have all but disappeared from the scene.

CCD cameras have good resolution but less sensitivity than that of the tube camera. The MOS cameras have even better resolution, but at the expense of still less sensitivity. Technologic breakthroughs in semiconductor manufacturing have brought the sensitivity of current CCD cameras close to that of the tube camera. They are therefore the most widely used type of camera today. On average, their sensitivity is of the order of 10 lux (a lux is a unit of sensitivity for electronic optical sensors). We use a CCD camera with 5-lux sensitivity and a resolution of 240,000 pixels.

Future technologic innovations will undoubtedly continue to improve cameras by making them smaller, more sensitive, and with better resolution.

The sensitivity of photographic film depends on the type of photochemical emulsions used. This sensitivity is measured by the film's ASA number, which represents the speed with which the emulsion reacts to light. There are films having an ASA number as high as 1600, allowing photography without a flash. However, resolution is better with a 200 ASA emulsion and flash illumination.

Image size

The larger the area covered by the image, the more light energy is needed to record it. This fact is of relatively limited importance in video recording. In photography using 35-mm film (standard slides), the exposed plate is approximately 90 times larger than for an 8-mm video camera. This enormous difference explains the necessity for a flash.

Recording equipment

Video cameras usually have a fixed focus, adapted for use with endoscopes. The electronic standards are PAL and SECAM in Europe and NTSC in the United States. Obviously both camera and recorder must "speak the same language" electronically. There are a variety of tape formats (Table 4.1), some more expensive than others. In general, the wider tapes are more sensitive than narrower ones. Here also technology is making giant steps forward, both in reducing the size of the tape and increasing its resolution.

TABLE 4.1 **Advantages and disadvantages of various video systems**

Format	Advantages	Disadvantages

8 mm	Compact
	Good resolution
	Editing unit available
	  at low cost and
	  user-friendly
	Small size of tapes
		Sound synchronization
		  difficult

VHS	Widespread availability Compact Affordable	Moderate quality Editing somewhat difficult Rapid loss of quality in dubbing
Super VHS	Excellent resolution	Incompatible with VHS Not widespread Expensive
UMATIC 3/4 inch	Excellent resolution Easy editing	Heavy equipment Expensive Cumbersome

Setting up the operating room

Setting up the equipment in the operating room ahead of time is essential to minimize problems and loss of time during video recording of a procedure.

Ideally, the monitor is fixed on the wall at the right side of the foot of the operating table. Two screens, one on the right and one on the left, are even better. Both operator and assistant, as well as the nurses and anesthetist, will then be able to observe the image unobstructed. In the absence of such a wall-mounted fixture, the monitor can be placed on top of a video cart.

The video cart must be extra sturdy but easily moved around the room. On the cart are
- The video recorder on the lowest level
- The camera and light source on the upper level

Manufacturers now offer factory-assembled units with integrated connections. These carts are rather expensive but extremely handy.

All elements of the video system depend on one another and contribute to the basic goal, which is obtaining a good-quality image—testimony of reality.

Recording and storage of images

Video monitoring is the acquisition of visual information.

We have explained why an image of the highest quality is of utmost importance. Let us now discuss the problems generated by recording and storage of these images.

Video recording

Continuous recording of an endosurgical intervention results in a rather lengthy, uncoordinated succession of images with long slack periods. To avoid this, two techniques are possible: editing and timed recording.

Editing requires the enlistment of professional technicians or the acquisition of expensive equipment and is therefore practical only for those individual physicians or institutions for whom finances are no consideration or when used only for specific, isolated events such as scientific meetings. Moreover, editing requires high-quality recording (e.g., with 3/4-inch systems), increasing the cost even more.

Timed recording is a real time technique that avoids editing. However, the entire operating team must adhere to a strict discipline. This is how it works: After initial visualization of the abdominal contents and after deciding what procedure will be performed, the surgeon records for a brief period of time to provide an overview of the pathology. Then, at intervals, short sequences are recorded pertaining to important aspects of the surgery. At the end of the procedure, another overview is recorded, as well as some closeup views of important areas in the surgical field. The operator may even wish to record an audio description of the procedure over a microphone onto the same tape. Timed recording saves editing time and money, while providing adequate visual documentation of good quality. Additionally, it forces the surgeon to be systematic in performing the procedure.

Storage

Storage of visual images rapidly becomes a problem. For optimal use of the recordings, one should establish and follow certain rules:

1) All cassettes must be properly labeled at the time of the operation (name, file number, diagnosis, surgery, time). It is a good idea to film the name tag of the patient prior to her surgery.

2) At regular intervals (ideally every week), the recordings should be reviewed and catalogued.

3) A log-book or, ideally, a computerized file system, must be updated daily.

4) All cassettes should be properly labeled. A good system is to use a six-digit number, of which the first four digits represent year and month (year-month-number).

5) Cassettes should be stored in a cool, dark, dry area.

These rules will promote optimal preservation and accessibility of the images.

Sterilization of equipment

Infection is a rare complication of laparoscopy. However, increased use of equipment such as video cameras could change this. All currently available models can be soaked in disinfecting solutions, but this all too frequently results in deposits on the lens and, in the long run, damages the camera.

Several techniques help keep the field sterile. Many surgeons use double gloves and allow the camera in the field only when all trocars are already in place. Having manipulated the camera, they then remove and discard the outer pair of gloves.

We favor using sterile, elastic gauze fitted around the camera and cable. Such "sleeves" are also available in plastic and are disposable—handy, but expensive.

Whatever technique is chosen, use of the camera increases the risk of contamination of the operative field.

A look to the future

The future in digital imaging is at our doorstep, represented by the optical laser disk, which already permits storage of a large number (1500/disk) of images, retrievable randomly at any time. Interest in this type of recording is based mainly on the interaction between computers and video images—the forthcoming mode for filing medical records.

Optical disks share many of the advantages of computer disks:
- Fast locating of a file
- long-distance transfer of images (via modem)
- User-friendly features

Current optical disks are impractical, because storage of images destroys the template, making them nonreusable. Sony Corporation recently developed a reusable disk based on a phtalocyanine coating with organic chromophores. These chromophores absorb light from a laser beam. The laser beam thus creates "spots" on the disk. However, these disks are of very low capacity—too low for the storage of sequences of video film. The disk can be erased only under conditions of specified temperature and humidity, and this wipes the entire disk clean.

Research is under way on disks having multiple layers of chromophores. Each layer would absorb a particular band of frequencies of light energy from a laser beam. This would permit storage of entire sequences of digitalized images combined with information from a computer. Moreover, selective erasing would be possible, permitting digital editing of video sequences. One may be sure that the coming years will bring a profound revolution in the storage of medical records, especially where endoscopic procedures are involved.

Conclusion

Video documentation and video-guided surgery are two new techniques engendered by technologic innovations of the last decade. It is foreseeable that this mutation will go on in the years to come and that by the end of the century our daily practice of medicine will have changed dramatically. We have to take responsibility for shaping the future by answering these two questions honestly:

- Which technologic advances profit the patient and her physician?
- How should we as physicians prepare ourselves so as to be able to utilize these technologic innovations?

5

Anesthesia

P. Schoeffler, C. Henry, and C. Monteillard

The last few years have brought two major changes to laparoscopy:
- Expansion of indications
- Increasingly complex surgery

The prolonged duration of the procedures imposes an additional burden on the anesthesiologist to correct for insufflation of large volumes of CO_2 and prolonged Trendelenburg position. A good understanding of the physiologic changes is therefore required. This chapter will begin with a description of the pathophysiologic changes, followed by a discussion of the various modalities of anesthesia available.

Pathophysiology

Respiratory changes (Fig. 5.1)

CO_2 is a gas that diffuses readily within the tissues, reducing the risk of gas embolism in case of accidental intravascular injection. The high diffusion constant of CO_2 also leads to peritoneal absorption, resulting in hypercapnia— a fact that has been emphasized in the literature [15–17]. In patients on

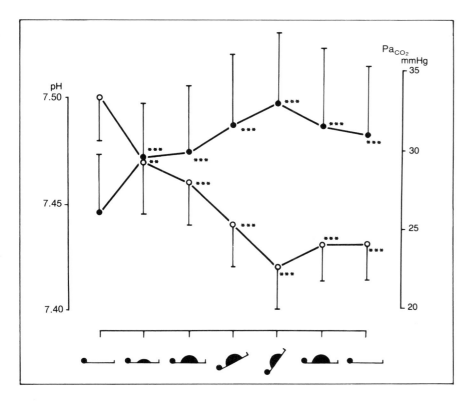

5.1 Changes in arterial pH and Pa_{CO_2} during insufflation (15 and 30 cmH$_2$O) and during Trendelenburg position (15 and 30°). Bars indicate the standard deviation. Statistical analysis is calculated in relation to the initial, preoperative values: * = $p < 0.05$; ** = $p < 0.01$; *** = $p < 0.001$. (With permission from Schoeffler et al. [15].)

curarimimetic agents and artificial ventilation, an additional factor presents itself: diaphragmatic motion is altered, as described by Froese and Byran [6]. The posterior portion of the diaphragm is less well mobilized by ventilation and thereby alters the ventilation-perfusion ratio. The dorsal pulmonary lobes are well perfused but not well ventilated, and, conversely, the ventral lobes are well ventilated but less well perfused in the dorsal decubitus position. This alteration in ventilation-perfusion ratio leads to an increased *shunt effect* in the posterior lobes and increased *dead space* in the anterior lobes. The latter enhances the rise in Pa_{CO_2}. Trendelenburg positioning exacerbates these changes.

In addition, the pneumoperitoneum leads to displacement of the endotracheal tube, with risk of selective right lung ventilation, resulting in left atelectasis. The endotracheal tube should be well positioned, fixed with care, and ventilation checked whenever the position of the patient is changed [14].

Cardiovascular changes (Fig. 5.2)

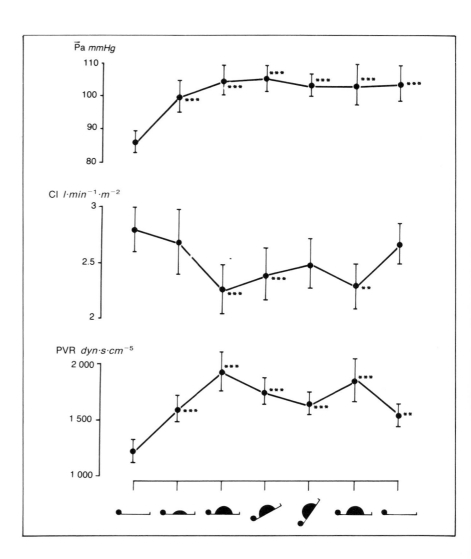

5.2 Changes in mean arterial pressure ($\bar{P}a$), cardiac index (CI) and peripheral vascular resistance (PVR) during peritoneal insufflation (15 and 30 cmH$_2$O) and Trendelenburg position (15 and 30°). Values given are the mean and standard deviation. Statistical analysis is calculated in relation to the initial preoperative values: $^* = p < 0.05$; $^{**} = p < 0.01$; $^{***} = p < 0.001$. (With permission from Schoeffler et al. [15].)

The cardiovascular changes observed during laparoscopy represent the combined effects of the pneumoperitoneum and the Trendelenburg position. During insufflation, when intra-abdominal pressure reaches $30 \, cmH_2O$, the cardiac output decreases $\pm 20 \%$ [15]. Other investigators [12] have also observed a linear relationship between reduction of cardiac output and increase in intra-abdominal pressure. The pathophysiology of this phenomenon is not entirely clear. One may assume that decrease in cardiac output is related to reduction in venous return from the lower extremities, a result of compression of the intra-abdominal large vessels [13]. This reduction in venous return, however, is not paralleled by a reduction in cardiac end-diastolic pressure. Indeed, right atrial and pulmonary capillary pressures are elevated [15]. This apparent contradiction is due to increased thoracic pressure during intra-abdominal insufflation.

Increased peripheral vascular resistance can be explained at least partially by intra-abdominal compression of the large vessels [9, 10, 12, 13]. During Trendelenburg positioning, the cardiac output increases slightly [15]. This is probably due to a temporary increase in venous return. The latter phenomenon, however, does not completely reverse the decrease in cardiac output caused by the pneumoperitoneum.

Gastrointestinal changes

Increased intra-abdominal pressure and Trendelenburg positioning both favor gastric reflux. The use of an endotracheal tube with an inflatable balloon is therefore recommended. Irritation of the peritoneum at the level of the diaphragm, due to residual CO_2 gas, causes referred pain in the right shoulder, because of C4 metameric innervation of the diaphragm.

Anesthetic techniques

General anesthesia

General anesthesia was long the only technique used for laparoscopy. It remains the one most utilized and requires strict adherence to a specific protocol. Patients are usually young and in good health, hospitalized for benign pathology. All accidents and, a priori, those related to anesthesia, are truly dramatic. Moreover, the increase in lengthy endosurgical interventions requires a well thought out technique.

Preoperative assessment aims at detecting the common contraindications for endoscopy: chronic heart failure and intracranial hypertension. Prior spontaneous pneumothorax and/or pulmonary emphysema should also lead to increased caution. Obesity, without repercussion on respiratory or cardiovascular states, is not a contraindication for anesthesia [15]. However, obesity may lead to increased technical difficulties, especially in establishing the pneumoperitoneum. A complete physical examination requiring no additional tests is generally sufficient in the young female with a negative history.

Administration of premedication varies from one school of thought to another. Vagolytic agents are no longer required when using the latest anesthetic drugs, which do not induce bradycardia or bronchial hypersecretion. Anxiolytic agents (usually of the benzodiazepine family) are indicated in anxious patients. Such drugs are being increasingly administered orally rather than intramuscularly, as the latter route is painful and shows a lower bioavailablity. Other drugs, such as hydroxyzine (Atarax), are useful in patients with allergies because of their antihistaminic effect (H_1 receptor blockage).

Cardiac monitoring is mandatory during all laparoscopies. Use of the CM5 lead allows detection of a potential repolarization anomaly. Because of important cardiovascular fluctuations, it is advisable to use an automatic blood pressure cuff for readings at regular intervals. A large-caliber venous access is important for rapid fluid replacement, should this be required.

The classic lithotomy position induces unfavorable cardiovascular changes, especially at the end of the procedure, when the legs of the patient are lowered. In case of hypovolemia, venous pooling in the lower extremities causes reduction of venous return and a fall in arterial pressure. The classic lithotomy position also leads to compression lesions of the nervus peroneus communis if the legs are improperly positioned in the stirrups. Many physicians prefer the dorsal decubitus position with legs apart, a position that allows equal if not increased comfort for the surgeon.

A shoulder support is used routinely, but it must be correctly positioned at the level of the acromion, so as to avoid injury to the brachial plexus. The arm having intravenous access should be fixed to an arm rest; the other arm should be positioned alongside the patient, restrained by a towel, the ends of which are tucked underneath the patient, instead of using braces. These may cause injury, especially during prolonged surgery [14].

Induction of anesthesia starts with denitrogenization through ventilation with pure oxygen for 3 to 5 min. The choice of drug depends on the projected length of the anesthesia or on any possible allergies of the patient. When the intervention is projected to be of short duration, an anesthetic agent having a short half-life, such as propofol, should be used. Allergies of the patient may require the use of drugs having a low histamine-releasing effect, such as midazolam or etomidate. Endotracheal intubation is mandatory. This is facilitated by use of depolarizing curarimimetic drugs such as suxamethonium. However, because of the relatively high stimulatory effect on histamine release, many anesthesiologists prefer to use a nondepolarizing curare agent, sometimes adding a so-called priming agent to shorten the latency period of these drugs. One must emphasize, at this point, the importance of good communication between anesthetist and surgeon. Nondepolarizing curarimimetic drugs cause prolonged muscle relaxation, especially of the abdominal wall. This may come as a surprise to a surgeon who is accustomed to introducing needles and trocars through a relatively tonic abdominal wall. Intubation permits assisted ventilation. Slight hyperventilation corrects the hypercapnia caused by absorption of CO_2 through the peritoneum.

Anesthesia is maintained by a mixture of oxygen and nitrous oxide. Gas analysis shows that a 50% oxygen content at inspiration is sufficient to maintain correct oxygenation. Gas anesthetic agents such as halothane, enflurane, and isoflurane potentiate the anesthetic effects of nitrous oxide. We must remember, however, that halothane and enflurane lower the cardiac output, and all three gases cause a redistribution of the systemic circulation, lowering perfusion of the mesenteric vessels. This may add to the negative effects of increased intra-abdominal pressure, especially during prolonged interventions. The effects of these gases on intracranial pressure must be considered, especially because of the Trendelenburg position.

The use of systemic analgesics is widespread. Their use permits reduction of autonomic nervous reactions to painful stimuli and potentiates the effect of hypnotic drugs. However, laparoscopy usually induces less pain than does open surgery, especially in the postoperative phase, and less medication is therefore required—an important point, as the residual effect of systemic analgesics may lead to unnecessary postoperative respiratory depression. For this reason also, short-acting drugs, such as fentanyl or, better, alfentanil, are preferred. If necessary, the action of morphinomimetics can be reversed by naloxone. In all cases, postoperative surveillance by qualified personnel in a well-equipped area is desirable. During prolonged interventions, intra-abdominal hyperpressure can be limited by using curarimimetic agents, which will facilitate venous return and reduce ventilation pressure. It is advisable to monitor paralysis with electric nerve stimulation.

Waking the patient is as important as inducing anesthesia: Trendelenburg should be reversed before the pneumoperitoneum is released. Evacuation of CO_2 should be as complete as possible, to reduce postoperative shoulder pain. In addition, vital signs should be monitored at frequent intervals. Spontaneous respiration and a return to normal consciousness should precede extubation. Even when the patient is wide awake, surveillance in a recovery area is mandatory, especially if morphinomimetic drugs have been used.

Postoperative recovery is usually short. Food and liquid ingestion is possible within a few hours following extubation, so that venous access is no longer required. Postoperative pain is moderate and, in general, requires no systemic analgesics. The brevity of the postoperative recovery period has led to the widespread use of laparoscopy on an outpatient basis [14]. At our institution, we consider ambulatory surgery only in simple procedures (e.g., sterilization) and only under ideal circumstances (help at home, living near the hospital, etc.).

Alternative techniques

Local anesthesia, with or without paracervical block, is used by certain teams on a large scale [2, 3, 11] for short interventions, e.g., sterilization or oocyte retrieval. The chief advantages of this technique are its low cost and simplicity. One may be tempted, for added patient comfort, to combine local anesthesia with tranquilizers or systemic analgesics. However, the respiratory depression caused by these drugs could exacerbate the hypercapnia caused by CO_2 absorption. Reports in the literature [11] suggest a beneficial effect in lowering postoperative pain by injection of bupivacaine into the broad ligament prior to sterilization.

Epidural anesthesia seems to be preferable because, if properly placed (D6 or even D4), it provides sufficient analgesia. There have been studies reporting satisfactory results with the use of epidural anesthesia for outpatient surgery [4] and assisted reproductive techniques [7]. The authors report minimal variations in pulse, arterial pressure, and respiratory physiology (no significant hypercapnia, despite spontaneous ventilation). We refrain from recommending this technique as routine. Indeed, the data fail to report changes of cardiac output and end-diastolic pressure. One wonders what effects the pneumoperitoneum, combined with a sympathetic block, have on venous return. Moreover, an epidural block at D4 interferes with cardiac innervation, eliminating reflex tachycardia in case of sudden hypotension.

Conclusion

Anesthesia has been forced to keep up with the extraordinary evolution of laparoscopy over the past two decades. Safety of the patient is the main objective. The liberal use of endoscopic interventions necessitates a definition of standards for the surgeon as well as for the anesthetist.

References

1. Alexander C.D., Wetchler B.V., Thompson R.E., « Bupivacaine infiltration of the mesosalpinx in ambulatory surgical laparoscopic tubal sterilization », *Can. J. Anaesth.*, 1987; 34 : 362-365.
2. Audra Ph., Dargent D., « La stérilisation per-cœlioscopique sous anesthésie locale », *Fertil. Steril.*, 1984; 12 : 943-945.
3. Belaisch J.C., Guillet-Rosso F., Baton C., Champagne C., Bodereau A.M., Frydman R., « Cœlioscopie sous anesthésie locale pour recueil d'ovocytes en vue d'une fécondation in vitro », *Presse Méd.*, 1983; 23 : 2053-2054.
4. Bridenbaugh L.D., Soderstrom R.M., « Lumbar epidural block anesthesia for out-patient laparoscopy », *J. Reprod. Med.*, 1979; 23 : 85-86.
5. Brown J.R., Fishburne J.I., Roberson V. et al., « Ventilatory and blood gas changes during laparoscopy with local anesthesia », *Am. J. Obstet. Gynecol.*, 1976; 124 : 741-745.
6. Froese A.B., Bryan A.C., « Effects of anesthesia and paralysis on diaphragmatic mechanics in man », *Anesthesiology*, 1974; 41 : 242-255.
7. Gouezel H., Boulbin J., Faucheux M., Saout H., Legrand G., Lebervet J.Y., Malledant Y., Saint-Marc C., « Anesthésie péridurale pour la fécondation in vitro et la transplantation embryonnaire sous cœlioscopie », *Cah. Anesthesiol.*, 1987; 35 : 611-616.
8. Haberer J.P., Bouetard E., Jacquetin J., « Examen pré-anesthésique: examens à pratiquer, médicaments à interrompre », (pp. 305-330). In: Résumés des Communications. MAPAR Ed., Paris, 1985.
9. Ivankovich A.D., Miletich D.J., Albrecht R.F., Heyman H.J., Bonnet R.F., « Cardiovascular effects of intraperitoneal insufflation with carbon dioxide and nitrous oxide in the dog », *Anesthesiology*, 1975; 42 : 281-287.
10. Lenz R.J., Thomas T.A., Wilkins D.G., « Cardiovascular changes during laparoscopy », *Anaesthesia*, 1976; 31 : 4-12.
11. Mackenzie I.Z., Turner E., O'Sullivan G.M., Guillebaud J., « Two out-patient laparoscopic clip sterilizations using local anesthesia », *Br. J. Obstet. Gynaecol.*, 1987; 94 : 449-453.
12. Marshall R.L., Jepson P.J.R., Davie I.T., Scott D.B., « Circulatory effects of carbon dioxide insufflation on the peritoneal cavity for laparoscopy », *Br. J. Anesth.*, 1972; 44 : 680-684.
13. Marshall R.L., Jepson P.J.R., Davie I.T., Scott D.B., « Circulatory effects of peritoneal insufflation with nitrous oxide », *Br. J. Anaesth.*, 1972; 44 : 1183-1187.
14. Prentice J.A., « The Trendelenburg position, Anesthesiologic considerations. In Positioning in Anesthesia and Surgery », (pp. 98-114). J.T. Martin Ed., Saunders, Philadephia, 1978.
15. Schoeffler P., Haberer J.P., Manhes H., Henry C., Habouzit J.L., « Répercussions circulatoires et ventilatoires de la cœlioscopie chez l'obèse », *Ann. Fr. Anesth. Réanim*, 1984; 3 : 10-15.
16. Souron R., Nicolas F., « Etude expérimentale des mécanismes d'augmentation de la $PaCO_2$ au cours des cœlioscopies » *Anesth. Analg.*, 1973; 30 : 493-501.
17. Souron R., Nicolas F., « Etude des gaz du sang au cours des cœlioscopies comportant la réalisation de pneumopéritoine au CO_2 » *Anesth. Analg.*, 1973; 30 : 506-511.

6

Complications

For a long time, laparoscopy was considered a dangerous procedure. In 1976, Mintz [1, 2] reported 194 complications, including 19 deaths, in 100,000 laparoscopies. In his introduction, Mintz stated: "Don't look for explanations; it is not the celioscopy, it is the celioscopist." As proof of his statement, the Club des Celioscopistes Français [5] published a report of 13 emergency laparotomies for complications in 9682 celioscopies, with no mortalities. The main difference between these two statistics is the level of expertise of the surgeon. The first report was based on a nationwide survey; the second represents data from a small number of experienced endoscopists. This chapter deals with accidents related to surgical intervention; anesthesia-related problems are discussed in Chapter 5.

Complications in general

Establishing the pneumoperitoneum and introducing the trocar are truly blind procedures. Accidents therefore occur, especially if an improper method was used (see Chapter 2).

Sound technique reduces the likelihood of complications.

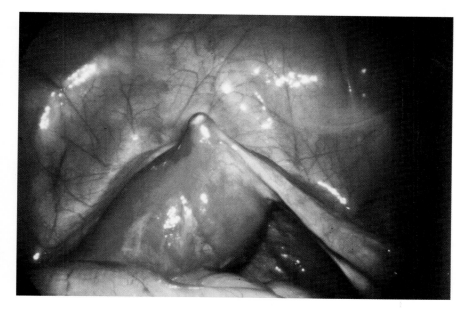

6.1 Uterine perforation. This is a minor complication and in general does not require any treatment. To avoid this complication, it is advisable not to use the hysterometer for manipulation of the uterus, a maneuver which can sometimes involve quite some force.

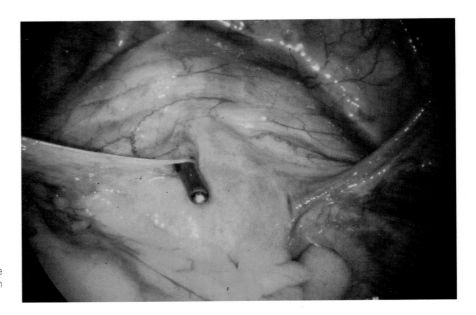

6.2 Use of Hegar probes does not preclude the occurrence of perforation. A Hegar probe is seen piercing the vesicouterine fold.

Complications related to establishing the pneumoperitoneum

During insertion, the Verres needle can injure any intra-abdominal organ, vessel, or the omentum. The complication will be recognized either immediately (blood spurting out of the needle), shortly thereafter (aspiration of bowel contents), or eventually (high end-insufflation pressure). Whatever the scenario, the needle should simply be removed and gently reinserted. Pneumoperitoneum is then established, and the abdominal contents are carefully inspected. Laparotomy is indicated only if there is a sudden change in the hemodynamic status of the patient, indicating severe hemorrhage.

How can one avoid these complications? Establishing the pneumoperitoneum is certainly the most difficult part of the procedure, because it is a completely blind maneuver. Three fundamental rules can lower the risk of complications:

– Choose a site of insertion away from existing scars.

– Elevate the abdominal wall to increase the distance between it and the great vessels.

– Introduce the needle no farther once it is perceived that the peritoneal cavity has been entered.

When performed correctly, establishment of the pneumoperitoneum gives rise to only minor complications, such as emphysema of the omentum or retroperitoneal space (Figs. 6.3, 6.4, 6.5). The use of an automatic insufflator lowers this risk. Indeed, the machine will "refuse" to insufflate except when the needle is located in a space having low resistance.

Minor injuries to the epigastric vessels, caused by the Verres needle or suprapubic trocar, are relatively frequent but without consequence. They can be avoided by intraumbilical insufflation and insertion of the suprapubic trocar medially from the umbilical ligaments. In case of such an injury, the skin is incised below the trocar (± 2 cm) and a ligature applied with a Deschamps needle under visual control, thereby avoiding laparotomy.

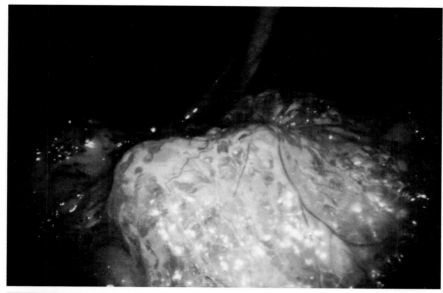

6.3 Emphysema of the omentum is a minor complication. It occurs more often when the needle is not sharp because more force is needed to pierce the abdominal wall.

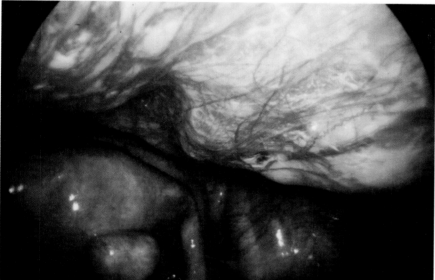

Follow two examples of retroperitoneal emphysema of the abdominal wall

6.4 Retroperitoneal emphysema of the anterior abdominal wall is a common complication of the novice laparoscopist who—excessively prudent—inserts the needle too tangentially.

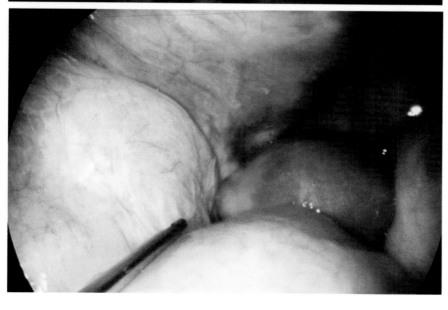

6.5 Retroperitoneal emphysema of the posterior wall is more worrisome because of the vital structures involved. This complication should spur the surgeon to review his method of insertion of the needle. Insertion into the vena cava or the iliac vein is rare but not exceptional.

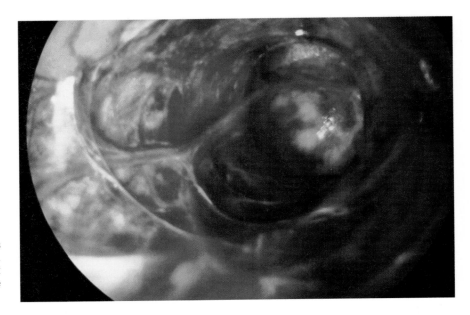

6.6 Fausse route of the first-puncture trocar is caused by introduction with too steep an angle. The space of Retzius is entered, which does not present any problems, as demonstrated by the technique of retroperitoneoscopy.

Complications related to the first-puncture trocar

Such injuries are uncommon but dramatic. Injuries of the aorta and vena cava lead to severe, sometimes lethal hemorrhage requiring immediate laparotomy for hemostasis. One should, in such a case, also consider the risk of gas emboli. All bowel injuries require immediate laparotomy for repair.

How can one avoid these complications? Again, prevention is based upon three simple rules:

– Insert the trocar only if the pneumoperitoneum has been properly established. There is no golden rule as to how much gas should be insufflated or how high the intra-abdominal pressure should be. The trocar should be introduced only when the abdominal wall is felt to be well distended and offers sufficient resistance to the trocar, which can be easily perceived by the experienced endoscopist via palpation.

– Choose an insertion site in an area free of adhesions. The umbilical area is the obvious choice. However, when the abdominal wall bears a lower midline scar, insertion can be performed at another site.

– Terminate the procedure if no zone free of adhesions is located. This zone should be at least 5 cm in diameter.

Complications of laparoscopic surgery

Bowel injury

Bowel injury is not unusual when extensive adhesiolysis or treatment of pelvic abscesses is undertaken laparoscopically. Most important is prompt recognition and treatment, usually by laparotomy. The really serious complications occur when the injury goes unnoticed [4], resulting in peritonitis. Moreover, the initial symptoms of such injuries are often lost among the "usual postoperative complaints," leading to relatively late diagnosis of the condition. This set of circumstances represents the major cause of morbidity, even mortality, due to laparoscopy. Prevention consists of applying a standardized technique and systematically inspecting the bowel following adhesiolysis to detect any inadvertent injury that may have occurred during surgery.

Hemorrhage

Complications vary according to whether the hemorrhage occurs immediately or later on. The risk of hemostasis is related to

– The method employed: risks due to use of monopolar coagulation or injection of vasopressin.

– The time required to achieve hemostasis: injury of the infundibulopelvic ligament can be treated at laparoscopy if the surgeon and the entire operating team move swiftly. If, within 2 to 3 min, hemostasis is not achieved, it is advisable to proceed with laparotomy rather than desperately continue to coagulate and coagulate, which then becomes quite hazardous.

Incomplete hemostasis leads to delayed bleeding or to slow development of a hematocele. The latter can be evacuated at a second laparoscopy if one wishes to lower the risk of infection and adhesion formation. When hemostasis, especially of large areas, is uncertain, one can insert a drain (Redon drain), which will avoid the formation of a hematocele and assure early diagnosis of delayed bleeding.

Electrosurgical burn

Electrical burn is a feared complication, because its perception is usually delayed. Indeed, the burn may occur at a distance from the site of application. The necrotic site will slough within 8 to 9 days and lead to perforation with secondary peritonitis. These accidents usually occur with defective instrumentation (damaged insulation) or by inadvertent activation of the foot pedal. They are therefore avoidable.

- Limit the use of monopolar coagulation to easily accessible sites.
- Disconnect the instrument as soon as it is no longer being used.
- Use only instruments with retractable electrodes.
- Check all instruments for defects at regular intervals.

The use of alternative coagulation techniques, in particular bipolar coagulation, is advisable.

Complications due to use of the laser

The laser is an excellent surgical instrument that is safe in well-trained hands. On the other hand, it becomes a dangerous tool when used by an inexperienced surgeon. A "lost shot" can cause damage at a distance, thus going unnoticed. Use of the laser should be prohibited except by those surgeons who have prior experience in both endoscopic techniques and use of the laser. Prevention of accidents lies in the use of instruments with backstop, in profuse use of fluid in the cul-de-sac, and in observing good surgical technique, such as operating only at a safe distance from the bowel.

Complications due to use of vasopressin (POR 8)

Vasopressin has brought an undeniable advantage to endosurgery. Risks secondary to its use are, however, severe. Vasopressin is a potent vasoconstrictor, a property that can lead to hypertensive crises and severe vasoconstriction of the coronary arteries. In our experience, we have observed only one case of acute pulmonary edema 4 h after injection. The cause-and-effect relationship could not be fully established. Prevention lies in correct extravascular injection of the drug, diluted to 1 IU:4 to 8 mL of physiologic solution. (Note: the potency of POR 8 is greater than that of Pitressin.) Use of chemical hemostasis should be limited to a minimum. Its use is most effective in the treatment of ectopic pregnancy. Indeed, the vessels of the mesosalpinx are readily recognized and risk of intravascular injection is therefore reduced. The anesthetist should be informed prior to injection of POR 8, in order to monitor more closely hemodynamic changes and to request discontinuation of the injection should that be necessary.

Other complications

The bladder can be punctured with the suprapubic trocar, especially if there is a scar from a previous laparotomy. If such an injury goes unnoticed, it can lead to urinary peritonitis, a very serious complication. Treatment consists of installing an indwelling catheter in the bladder for ± 8 days and intraperitoneal drainage (for detection of a leak) for 48 h. If leakage occurs, the defect must be surgically closed.

The fallopian tube can be transected during adhesiolysis, especially when pelvic inflammatory disease is present or during attempted extraction of an instrument still clamped onto the oviduct. Hemostasis can be obtained by using vasopressin injected into the mesosalpinx or by bipolar coagulation. The problem of tubal reconstructive surgery should be discussed on a case-by-case basis.

Conclusion

History has taught us that observance of standardized and safe maneuvers and a thorough acquaintance with contraindications limit the occurrence of complications. Therefore, all surgeons, even the most experienced, should "stick to the rules."

References

1. Mintz M., « Le risque et la prophylaxie des accidents en cœlioscopie gynécologique: enquête sur 100 000 cas », *J. Gynécol. Obstet. Biol. Reprod.*, 1976; 5 : 681-695.
2. Mintz M., « Les accidents de la cœlioscopie et leur prophylaxie », *Con. Fert. Sex.*, 1984; 12 : 927-928.
3. Pierre F., « Le risque de plainte en responsabilité médicale dans la pratique chirurgicale gynécologique », Thèse, Clinique Gynécologique, Tours, 1987; 260.
4. Ravina J.H., Madelenat P., « Plaies viscérales et vasculaires ou cours de la cœlioscopie d'exploration: causes, responsabilité, prévention », *Con. Fert. Sex.*, 1984; 12 : 929-930.
5. Suchet J.H., Grumbach J.T., Loysel T., « Complication des œlioscopies colligées par le club gynéco-informatique en 1980–1982 », *Con. Fert. Sex.*, 1984; 12 : 901-903.

7
The laser

The laser was first channeled through an endoscope in our institution. Since then, we have observed a tremendous expansion of its use, especially in the United States. Endosurgical procedures are indeed the ideal type of intervention for use of the laser.

The CO_2 laser presents many advantages, among them the combination of different tissue effects using a single instrument: section of adhesions, vaporization of endometriotic nodules, or superficial coagulation. The laser beam can be tuned and modified in many different ways, allowing for the variety in tissue effects, from cutting to coagulation. For intelligent use of the laser, the surgeon is mandated to master the basics of optical physics, although this is not an exciting experience.

Biophysics of lasers [1]

What is a laser?

A laser emits a light beam that is unidirectional, monochromatic, and coherent. This means that all photons have the same wavelength and, therefore, the same energy, direction of propagation, and vibrational phase. In contrast, an incandescent or fluorescent light emits photons of variable wavelengths in all directions and phases. Monochromatic light is relatively easy to manipulate physically, because there is no diffraction phenomenon when entering a medium of different optical density. This allows the beam to be condensed into a very small area, increasing the energy at impact. The energy of conventional light diverges in all directions (it has a spherical distribution), which is mathematically represented by the steradian. The energy of an unfocused laser beam diverges over only a portion of a sphere, approximately 10^{-6} sr. Thus, for equal power output at the source, the energy at any distance from the source will be approximately $6 \cdot 10^6$ times higher with the laser source. Because laser light is usually converged into a small area, this difference is, in essence, much higher. Energy transfer is expressed in power density (W/cm^2) corresponding to energy per unit of surface.

Different types of lasers

There are many lasers, ranging from the low-power (milliwatts) laser in the supermarket to the high-power lasers of "Star Wars" (10^5 W). Each is characterized by its emission spectrum and power output.

In surgery, three lasers are commonly used: neodymium YAG (Nd:YAG), argon, and CO_2. Their number is likely to increase over the coming years. Each one has a particular wavelength: 10.6 nm for the CO_2 laser (far infrared), 1.06 nm for the Nd:YAG (infrared), and 0.437 for the argon (green). This results in some major differences.

– Argon and Nd:YAG lasers can be carried through optical fibers; CO_2 laser light cannot.

– CO_2 laser is immediately absorbed by water—argon much less so, and Nd:YAG even less than argon.

A new laser has recently entered the scene—the KTP-532—which can be used through optical fibers. Its characteristics are intermediate between those of the Nd:YAG and the CO_2 lasers [6].

Bioeffect of lasers [1, 3]

The laser transfers its energy to the tissue, causing a temperature increase. This thermodynamic effect depends on the amount of energy transmitted per unit of tissue volume. This depends on two variables: the power density at impact and the depth of penetration of the energy before it is completely absorbed. The following is a simplified example: A beam with a power density of 10,000 W/cm^2 will be absorbed within 0.01 cm (CO_2 laser), 0.4 cm (argon laser), and 3 cm (Nd:YAG laser). Per unit of tissue volume, therefore, the energy density will be 1×10^6 W/cm^3 for the CO_2, 25×10^3 for the argon, and 3.3×10^3 for the YAG laser. This, of course, is an approximation, because light absorption is a geometrical rather than a linear phenomenon.

Such a wide variety in energy concentration will obviously lead to various tissue effects. Three different effects are of interest:

– Vaporization (or section) occurs when absorption of energy is highly dense. The generated heat boils the intracellular water. Cells explode, emitting cellular debris and water vapor. Vaporization occurs within a small volume. This effect can be used to destroy abnormal tissue (e.g., endometriotic implants), to section adhesions, or to incise a hydrosalpinx.

– Coagulation occurs when the temperature within the tissue reaches 55° to 100° C. Cells are destroyed by denaturation of the proteins. In addition, small vessels (0.5 mm diameter in the case of the CO_2 laser) are obliterated.

– Reversible thermal damage occurs when the temperature does not reach 55° C. Cells are not destroyed and repair occurs readily, which may explain the phenomenon of rapid healing following use of the laser.

Practically all phenomena occur when the laser hits the tissue. Tissue is vaporized, and the generated heat causes coagulation and reversible damage at varying levels beneath the impact. The coagulation zone ensures hemostasis, which explains why the use of the laser is relatively bloodless. The relative dominance of these tissue effects depends on several factors: the wavelength of the laser, the power density, and the velocity of the beam.

• *Wavelength*. The CO_2 laser vaporizes better than it coagulates. The Nd:YAG laser vaporizes only minimally but coagulates extremely well. The argon laser performs somewhere in between. For each laser, coagulation is obtained at low power densities and vaporization at high power densities. The

CO_2 laser will require less power density (500 to 1000 W/cm^2) for cutting/vaporization than do the two others.

• *Power density.* Energy transfer is modulated by the spot size, which is determined by the focal length of the lens used and by the operator, who is able to focus or defocus the beam. A CO_2 laser at 10 W output will deliver 120×10^3 W/cm^2 when the spot size is 0.1 mm, 5×10^3 W/cm^2 when the spot size is 0.5 mm, and 0.3×10^3 W/cm^2 when the spot size is 2 mm. The effects are, respectively, cutting, vaporization, and coagulation.

• *Velocity.* This is an essential aspect when coagulation necrosis at the site of impact is considered. Indeed, the extent of coagulation necrosis is directly related to the duration of energy transfer. This explains why laser dissection should be done swiftly and why vaporization should be performed with sweeping movements, avoiding prolonged exposure at one site.

Bioeffects of the laser also depend on the composition of the tissue treated. The CO_2 laser will be more effective if the tissue contains a large amount of water. Argon is preferentially absorbed by hemoglobin and will cause coagulation more readily if the hemoglobin content of the tissue is high (e.g., endometriotic implants). This basic knowledge of laser physics is essential for understanding and using the laser in a competent manner.

CO_2 laser

The CO_2 laser is, practically speaking, the best adapted for use in gynecology. Coagulation is minimal but adequate for hemostasis of vessels 0.5 mm or less in diameter. The CO_2 laser can be used for superficial coagulation and is therefore extremely useful in tubal surgery; however, it can also be used for vaporization of such tissues as endometriotic implants. Use of the CO_2 laser in laparoscopy is not without difficulties, but it also has many potential benefits.

Limitations [4, 5, 10, 11]

There are five categories of limitations.

1) The CO_2 laser is not fiber-compatible. The beam is carried through an articulated arm—a cumbersome and heavy system. Moreover, it is not as easily manipulated as is a fiber system. Thus far, fiber systems for the CO_2 laser are not commercially available [2].

2) The laser probe must be airtight and connected to the CO_2 insufflator to avoid the deposition of particles on the lens.

3) The laser energy is partly absorbed by the CO_2 of the pneumoperitoneum [5].

4) The plume produced must be evacuated. Systems exist which ventilate the intra-abdominal area automatically when the laser is activated, but these are quite expensive.

5) The aiming beam (HeNe laser) is sometimes difficult to see because of the brightness of the light source. This effect is exaggerated when the beam is defocused.

Site of insertion [4, 9–11]

The ideal insertion site for the CO_2 laser was extensively discussed throughout the initial trials. Suprapubic access seemed most satisfactory but did not offer the safety of the coaxial mode of firing through the instrument channel of the endoscope. Our data have shown that suprapubic access offers more versatility and that the risks of "lost shots" have been greatly overestimated. Therefore we prefer this mode of access.

Argon laser [7]

We have no experience with this laser. Its major advantage is fiber compatibility. Another interesting characteristic is its preferential absorption by tissues rich in hemoglobin (e.g., endometriotic lesions). The argon laser can therefore be used to destroy endometriotic tissue in depth without bleeding or plume.

However, the disadvantages are multiple:

1) Section is not possible without coagulation, resulting in extensive tissue damage. The argon laser therefore cannot be used for microsurgical adhesiolysis, or a priori, for tubal reconstructive surgery.

2) Special protective eyewear is required.

3) The apparatus is very expensive.

Use of the argon laser seems to be limited to treatment of endometriosis. Even the early enthusiasts seem to agree that the future of the argon laser in laparoscopy is not all that bright.

Nd:YAG laser [8]

We have no experience with this type of laser either. Its principal advantage is its fiber compatibility. Its disadvantages are

1) Little cutting effect.

2) Deep penetration, which is a real danger in endosurgical applications.

The use of sapphire tips for focusing or defocusing may increase the usefulness of this laser in the future.

Indications

Endometriotic implants

The objective is destruction of lesions without damage to the surrounding tissues. The argon and Nd:YAG lasers can achieve this, but their relatively deep penetration is clearly a disadvantage. The CO_2 laser is the only one that permits accurate control of depth of destruction and is therefore extremely safe.

Endometriomas

Endometriomas should be removed by either endosurgery or minilaparotomy. When cystectomy seems technically difficult to perform, the base of the lesion can be vaporized with the CO_2 laser or coagulated with the YAG or argon lasers. This procedure is actually an acceptable indication for use of the fiber lasers.

Adnexal adhesiolysis

This is the ideal situation for use of the CO_2 laser, able to section the adhesions precisely and to vaporize the fibrin deposits on the ovarian surface. The CO_2 laser may be somewhat dangerous when dealing with type C adhesions, because the laser does not find the clevage plane as scissors do; rather, it creates one and therefore can injure organs involved in the adhesion process. The CO_2 laser should not be used in type C adhesions involving the bowel.

Tubal surgery

The tubal wall must be incised as sharply as possible. Among all available lasers, only the CO_2 lasers focus well enough to achieve this—for example, in ectopic pregnancy and neosalpingostomy.

Eversion of the tubal wall (salpingostomy) can be achieved with densities of less than 1000 W/cm^2 applied to the serosa. This superficial coagulation causes peritoneal retraction, resulting in eversion of the tube. Myomectomy, with or without prior treatment with LHRH agonists, is currently being evaluated. The capsule is incised with either CO_2 or YAG lasers and then the laser drills several tunnels within the myoma. This technique of myolysis needs further evaluation.

The future

Technologic advances in use of lasers in medicine will be multiple in the coming years, including:

– Wavelengths more suitable to surgery than the wavelength of the CO_2 laser

– Lasers with variable wavelengths, permitting a broader range of tissue effects

– More user-friendly equipment

– Lightweight, easy-to-use equipment with waveguides, which seem to us to be quite promising

– Defocusing systems which lessen the difficulties of locating the beam before firing [9]

Conclusion

Laser endoscopy started in our department in 1979. Its infancy was difficult, but now the progress is quite phenomenal, because the limits of endosurgery are once again being pushed forward. This technology will almost certainly surprise us with major changes in the coming years.

References

1. Baggish M., « Basic and advanced laser surgery in gynecology », Ed. Appleton-Century-Crofts, East Norwalk, Connecticut, 1985.
2. Baggish M., Elbakry M.M., « A flexible CO_2 laser fiber for operative laparoscopy », *Fertil. Steril.*, 1986; 46 : 16–20.
3. Beytout M., Mage G., Marquet C., Pouly J.L., Bruhat M.A., « Etude expérimentale de l'influence de puissance sur la vitesse de section et des lésions tissulaires en microchirurgie tubaire avec le laser CO_2 », *Laser Medical*, 81/82, ESI Pubilications, Masson, Paris, 1983; 11.
4. Bruhat M.A., Mage G., Manhes H., « Use of the CO_2 laser via laparoscopy. In: Laser Surgery III, Proceedings of the 3rd International Society for Laser Surgery », Ed. by I. Kaplan, Tel Aviv, International Society for Laser Surgery, 1979; 275.
5. Daniell J., Brown D., « CO_2 laser laparoscopy: initial experience in experimental animals and humans », *Obstet. Gynecol.*, 1982; 59 : 761.
6. Dorsey J., « Surgical treatment of endometriosis with the KTP 532 laser. Endometriosis », *Contr. Gynec. Obstet.*, 1987; 16 : 302.
7. Keye W.R., Dixon J., « Photocoagulation of endometriosis with the Argon laser through the laparoscope », *Obstet. Gynecol.*, 1983; 62 : 383.
8. Lomano J.M., « Photocoagulation of early pelvic endometriosis with the Nd:YAG laser through the laparoscope », *Laser Surgery Med.*, 1984; 3 : 328.
9. Nezhat C., Crowgey S.R., Garrisson C.P., « Surgical treatment of endometriosis via laser laparoscopy », *Fertil. Steril.*, 1986; 45 : 778–783.
10. Pouly J.L., Bruhat M.A., Mage G., Manhes H., « Utilisation du laser CO_2 par cœlioscopie: comparaison entre un branchement coaxial et un branchement sur trocar sus-pubien », *Acta. Med. Rom.*, 1982; 20 : 257–260.
11. Tadir Y., Kaplan I., Zuckerman Z., Edelsein T., Ovadia J., « New instrumentation and technique for laparoscopic CO_2 laser operations, a preliminary report », *Obstet. Gynecol.*, 1984; 63 : 582.

8

Pelvic inflammatory disease

Pelvic inflammatory disease (PID) is an emergency, both diagnostically and therapeutically.

Diagnostic laparoscopy

Although still considered controversial, laparoscopy is the obvious method of choice for the diagnosis of PID [6, 21, 42]. Physical examination and laboratory tests lead to a high incidence of false-positive and false-negative results, especially when dealing with the early stages of the disease [24]. However, it is precisely in the early stage, before clinical evidence presents itself, that therapy must be initiated if long-term complications are to be limited or avoided [34, 42–44]. In addition, laparoscopy offers more than mere diagnosis; it also permits a complete assessment of the pelvis and upper abdomen as well as initiation of treatment.

Prerequisites

Sampling of the endocervix for bacteriology

Sampling of the endocervix for bacteriology should be performed as the first step, especially in search of *Neisseria gonorrhoeae* or *Chlamydia trachomatis* [7, 22, 34].

Manipulation of the uterus

A hysterometer should not be used, as it leads all too frequently to uterine perforation and bleeding; it is better to use a Hegar probe or Cohen cannula. Initial manipulation of the uterus should be done under direct visualization. Adhesions to the posterior surface of the uterus are common and brisk manipulation can rupture them, resulting in bleeding, which will obscure the results of peritoneal cytology.

Suprapubic access

This is essential and can be done with either a blunt probe or an atraumatic forceps in the closed position.

Suction-rinsing apparatus

Frequent rinsing of the pelvic cavity is essential, especially when adhesiolysis causes diffuse oozing from the peritoneal surfaces.

Laparoscopic exploration

Exploration of the pelvis is preceded in all cases by sampling of the fluid in the cul-de-sac. This sampling is done for bacteriologic culture [7, 12, 23, 24, 40] but also for

    — A search for *Chlamydia* (culture or immunofluorescence with monoclonal antibodies) [12, 22, 39]. Abeille and Catalan proposed measuring anti-*Chlamydia* titers in the cul-de-sac fluid as a means of early and reliable diagnosis of acute salpingitis [1, 12].

    — Cytology, which allows more accuracy of diagnosis in the early stages, when the macroscopic aspect is still ambiguous [13, 30].

    — Measurement of substances such as orosomucoid, which is of interest in cases when the diagnosis is difficult [30].

It is mandatory to sample the liquid prior to manipulation of the organs, in order to avoid contamination with blood.

This is followed by complete inspection of the pelvis. The uterus is brought into extreme anteversion. The cul-de-sac is explored first. Obstructive adhesions should be divided to gain access. Next, each adnexa should be carefully inspected, first in overview, then in detail, by lifting the tube and ovary gently with a blunt instrument. Palpation of the tube is important in the early stages to evaluate the degree of edema and turgor of the tissue. Manipulation permits detection of peritubal adhesions and possible abscesses. Adhesiolysis and debridement of microabscesses are part of the evaluation of the extent of the disease. A distended tube, suspicious for pyosalpinx, should be punctured. At times, a simple "milking" of the tube will express pus from the lumen.

Visualization of the liver allows detection of perihepatic adhesions (Fitz-Hugh-Curtis syndrome [41]). The appendix and sigmoid must be carefully inspected; should the true culprit be appendicitis or diverticulitis, disastrous consequences could result [29]. Last but not least, when adhesions are present, a biopsy should be taken to confirm the presence of acute inflammation [25]. Intracellular inclusions, testimony to *Chlamydia* infection, can also be detected on histologic examination [44].

Classification

Pelvic inflammatory disease may be seen as a continuum of diseases, ranging from simple exudative salpingitis to ruptured pelvic abscess. This continuum is not linear and all intermediary steps are not obligatory. Although PID may present with many morphologic aspects, depending on the infectious agent and preexisting pelvic pathology [21, 29, 38, 40], it is convenient to divide the disease into three general stages by the most prominent sign of each stage: exudation, agglutination, and abscess formation. In each group, we will discuss the genital signs and peritoneal characteristics, which do not necessarily evolve simultaneously or in parallel [29, 32].

Exudation (Figs. 8.1 through 8.4)

Genital signs

Uterus and fallopian tubes present with edema and turgor. The mobility of the tube is reduced, especially in its isthmic portion. Vessels present an arachnoid aspect, due to vasodilation. Pressure on the tubes often causes turbid exudate to drip from the ampulla.

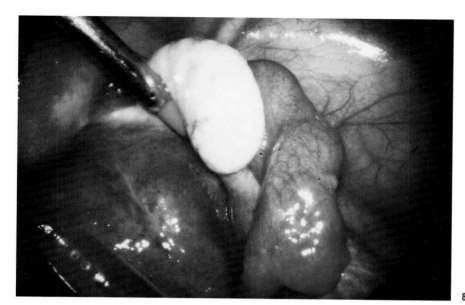

8.1 and 8.2 Acute salpingitis. The tube is reddened, edematous, and presents with vasodilatation.

8.1

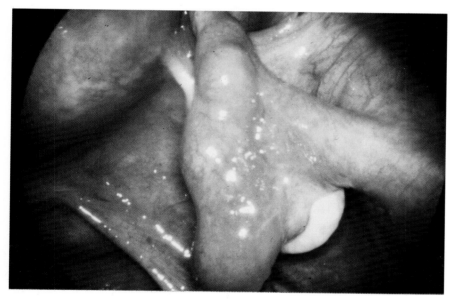

8.2

Peritoneal signs

The entire pelvis is involved in the inflammatory process. Four peritoneal signs can be discerned.
  – Mottled erythema.
  – Extremely reflective surfaces, caused by edema of the tissues.
  – Localized "tarnished" appearance of the peritoneum, especially at the level of the cul-de-sac. This may be considered a transitional stage between the exudative and agglutination phases of the disease.
  – Absence of excessive fluid; fluid present is turbid and rarely purulent. However, at times abundant purulent material may coexist with exudative salpingitis, especially in gonococcal infections.

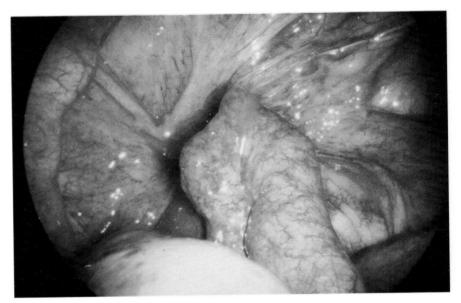

8.3 Later into the pathophysiology of the disease, changes of the tubal and parietal peritoneum are noted.

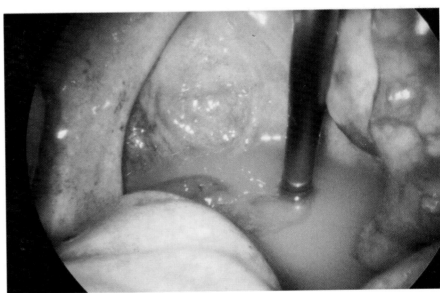

8.4 Pus collection in the cul-de-sac. Note the typical aspect of the peritoneum.

Agglutination (Figs. 8.5 through 8.7)

Genital signs

This is the stage of the *pachysalpinx*. The fallopian tube is thickened and rigid in all its segments; it appears increased in diameter and shortened. The mucosal folds of the fimbriae are edematous and agglutinated. Frequently pus may be seen dripping out of the tube.

Peritoneal signs

These signs are the most important at this stage of the disease. Mesothelial destruction leaves the surfaces raw, resulting in the agglutination of adjacent organs. At this point, the adhesions can easily be ruptured with a blunt probe and are either sticky, filmy deposits or veil-like and dotted with petechiae as a sign of ongoing infection.

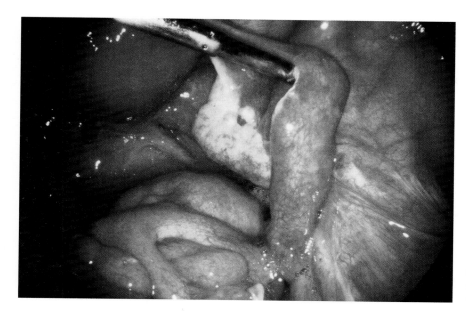

8.5 Agglutination stage. Using a probe, the surgeon detaches the tube from the ovary and demonstrates the presence of fibrinous deposits.

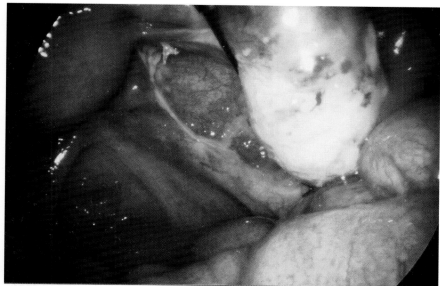

8.6 Aspect of the ovarian fossa (same patient as in 8.5).

Adhesions form through the proliferation of fibroblasts and macrophages and the eventual development of a vascular network (this type of adhesion appears at a later stage of development). Simultaneously, the extent of the adhesions increases, progressing from the fallopian tube to the ovary, the lateral wall and, finally, the cul-de-sac. Progressive isolation and partitioning of the cul-de-sac develop in a defense mechanism intended to avoid general peritonitis, and this leads to the next stage: abscess formation.

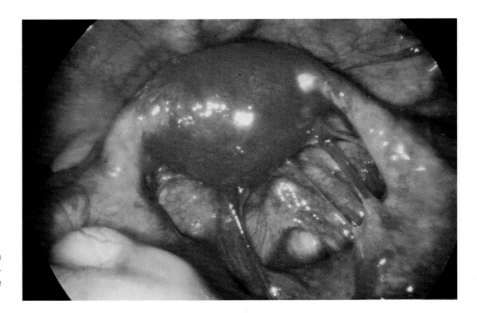

8.7 Another example of PID in the agglutination stage. Note the redness of the uterus, the vascularization of the adhesions, and the distortion of the isthmic portion of the left tube.

Abscess formation (Figs. 8.8 and 8.9)

Evolution toward abscess formation depends on the preexisting condition of the pelvis, the causative agent, and the latency period before diagnosis [5, 20, 26, 38].

True pyosalpinx

A true pyosalpinx is the result of a secondary infection of a hydrosalpinx. The tube is enlarged, reddened, and congested; the tubal wall is thickened and more rigid than that of the hydrosalpinx. Adhesions, if present, more likely represent sequelae from previous infectious episodes than part of the current process. The severity of the tubal inflammatory reaction is in marked contrast to the lack of peritoneal irritation; indeed, this discordance is highly suggestive of this diagnosis. Puncture, yielding pus, brings proof.

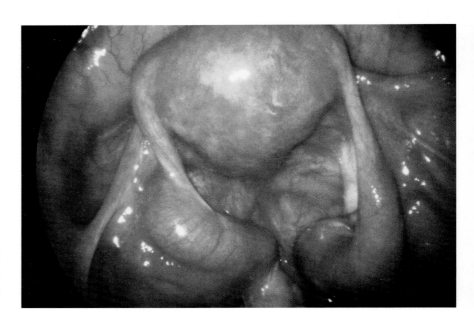

8.8 Bilateral pyosalpinx following hysterosalpingography. Note the striking absence of peritoneal irritation. The hypervascularization of the tubal wall distinguishes a pyosalpinx from a hydrosalpinx. In case of doubt, puncture of the tubal lumen is indicated.

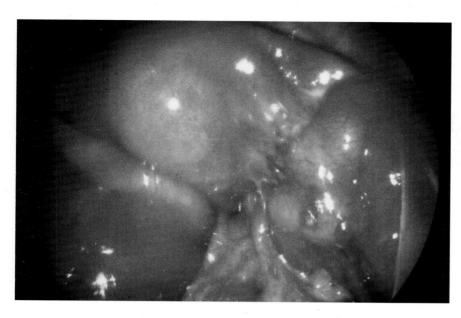

8.9 Pelvi-peritonitis. Involvement of the bowel adds a challenge to the endosurgical treatment. The oviducts are occluded and present with multiple small abscesses. Abscesses can also be found between tube and ovary, during dissection.

Tubal abscess resulting from recent occlusion

The macroscopic aspect is different from that of true pyosalpinx. The adnexae are enlarged and extremely edematous. The tube and ovary are involved in a conglomerate of adhesions with the posterior leaf of the broad ligament. Manipulation yields pus from pockets within the conglomerate. Gentle, blunt dissection often uncovers the fimbriated end of the tube and leads to positive diagnosis. The tube may spontaneously empty its purulent contents or else the operator is confronted with an occluded and abscessed tube. Two different mechanisms can lead to occlusion and abscess of the tube:

– The fimbriated end is caught up in adhesions with the posterior leaf of the broad ligament beneath the ovary or with the ovary itself. Mobilization of the oviduct therefore results in drainage of pus.

– The mucosal folds agglutinate and secondarily occlude the tube. Velamentous adhesions are easily recognized and can be removed by blunt dissection, resulting in drainage.

Tubo-ovarian abscess (TOA)

The adnexa is greatly enlarged, totally encapsulated, and often adherent to bowel and omentum. It becomes difficult to define the contours of the various organs within the mass. Gentle and extremely cautious adhesiolysis will progressively extricate oviduct and ovary.

Pus collection within the tube occurs frequently but not consistently. Two different entities must be considered [26]:

– *Recent TOA:* The adhesions encapsulating the adnexae create multiple small pockets of pus. Adhesiolysis is possible and allows identification of the organs, even though bowel may be involved. Simple inspection of the pelvis often underestimates the extent of the disease. Omitting the adhesiolysis in this case is a mistake, because microabscesses are left behind, and these are difficult to treat medically.

– *Chronic TOA:* Defined histologically as a heterogeneous mass, with some pus present; ovarian and tubal tissues can be recognized, with loss of well-defined boundaries. These lesions are impossible to treat conservatively by adhesiolysis. Often it is difficult to access the pelvis. This stage of the disease mandates laparotomy.

Abscess of the pouch of Douglas

This is the ultimate stage of PID. The diagnosis is a clinical one. Endoscopy reveals a complex mass filling the pelvis, with little chance to visualize the adnexae. Adhesiolysis and mobilization of the organs might possibly lead to a diagnosis, but involvement of often congested bowel segments demands extreme caution. Drainage by culdotomy is preferable as a first step.

Unusual presentations

Early or incompletely treated cases

Endoscopy reveals only minor changes such as a reddened appearance of the uterus and slight hyperemia of the tubes, which have, however, retained their normal suppleness. There is ample serous exudate in the cul-de-sac. Cytologic and bacteriologic evaluation of the exudate is the only method of diagnosing the infection. This often happens when antibiotic treatment was initiated prior to laparoscopy.

Subclinical or chronic cases [1, 25, 30, 33]

Minimal clinical signs and few macroscopic indications for an infectious process are the hallmarks of these cases. Again, diagnosis is made through cytology and bacteriology of the fluid in the cul-de-sac. These cases probably occur more often than is thought and may represent one reason for failure of microsurgical tubal reconstructive surgery–flareup of a preexisting infectious process puts a damper on the outcome of the surgery.

Cases associated with endometriosis

This association is quite unusual, as was reported by Schmidt [36] and later Forrest in a study in which routine bacteriologic examinations were performed on patients having endometriosis [16]. However, accurate diagnosis of early stages of the infection is difficult, because endometriosis also brings about an inflammatory reaction. Bacteriology of the cervix and peritoneal fluid is then the only differential criterion.

Misleading cases

Access to the pelvis may be difficult because of adhesions related to previous surgery, endometriosis, or an old infectious process. Adhesiolysis may be difficult and is therefore not recommended. The surgeon must decide, on a case-by-case basis, whether further exploration is warranted.

Rarely, acute inflammation may lead to hemoperitoneum. Thorough rinsing of the abdominal cavity will, however, quickly reveal the true etiology.

Bacteriology [5, 7, 15, 23, 24, 35, 38, 40, 43]

Polymicrobial infection of the oviduct and difficulty in identifying the infectious agents is due to the peculiar evolution of genital tract infection.

Typically, primary infection of the tube is due to bacteria of the STD type: *C. trachomatis, N. gonorrhoeae,* or perhaps *Mycoplasma.* The infection produces local changes such as impaired defense, disturbances in the physicochemical homeostasis of the oviduct, etc. These changes permit the development of secondary infection by bacteria from the intestinal or urinary tract: aerobic bacteria such as *Streptococcus, Staphylococcus*, or *Escherichia coli, Proteus*, etc. These bacteria accentuate the changes in the tubal milieu. The drop in pH and, above all, reduced oxygenation of the tissues lead to the appearance of anaerobic bacteria such as *Bacteroides fragilis*.

However, if preexisting tubal lesions, especially distal occlusion, are present, a second infectious episode can be initiated by an STD-type organism as well as a common saprophyte. Proof of this was provided by Daniell. Infectious complications of hysterosalpingography occur only in previously damaged tubes. Normal flora do not produce infection in a healthy tube; they can, however, colonize an abnormal oviduct.

The pathophysiology of acute salpingitis explains the difficulty of obtaining a definitive bacteriologic diagnosis and ensures a dilemma in the choice of appropriate antibiotics [11]. Identification of the pathogen is inconsistent. The yield depends on the quality and type of culture medium and on the proximity and expertise of the laboratory [23, 24]. A compromise must be sought between cost-effectiveness and performance. In our institution, we take five samples: a swab of the endocervix for culture of *Neisseria gonorrhoeae*, a Microtrack for *Chlamydia* identification, and samples on Schidler and IGV media in addition to blood samples for *Chlamydia* antibodies, which are taken at 20-day intervals. By following this protocol, we have reached an 80 % efficiency in detecting the causative organism [35].

Classifications

There are several classifications for acute salpingitis [21, 29]. None are really satisfactory: the COGIT (French study group) [21] classification is too complex, and the PID classification of Jacobson [29] too simplistic.

The classification we use takes the following factors into account: status of the oviduct, presence of TOA, presence of recent and/or preexisting adhesions. We discuss the importance of these factors later in this chapter.

Procedure

Adhesiolysis [9, 27, 34, 38] (Figs. 8.10, 8.11A, 8.11B, and 8.12)

Adhesiolysis is sometimes required in order to obtain a correct diagnosis, but it is also part of the treatment. The approach is the same as for adhesiolysis of old adhesions, namely:
   − From simple to complex
   − From inside to outside
The technique, as such, is different, however. The infected tissues are friable and tear easily, and this can create false surgical planes as well as causing irreparable damage. Therefore, the choice of instrument is extremely important. The blunt probe or atraumatic forceps in the closed position is the instrument of choice. Gentle mobilization of the adnexa is often enough to release the structures from the fibrinous exudate that has not yet organized into adhesions. Grasping of organs is to be avoided because, first of all, it is unnecessary, and second, because it can cause tubal or intestinal damage. If a firm grip should be required, it is advisable to grasp either the round or the ovarian ligament with a rounded atraumatic forceps.

The use of scissors is prohibited because, in addition to being of limited value, it is dangerous. The resection of recent adhesions is unnecessary—simple blunt dissection is all that is required. If the adhesion is a sequela of a past infection, surgical removal is not indicated, because recurrence is almost certain within the context of acute inflammation. Moreover, use of scissors for adhesiolysis will require manipulation of the tube and ovary, a maneuver not without risks, as outlined earlier. Freeing the bowel from an infected adnexa should be done only if the maneuver proceeds without difficulty. An abrupt movement by the surgeon presents a very real danger because of the lever effect: the force applied on the organs is higher than that exercised by the operator's hand. Adhesiolysis within an acutely infected pelvis requires strict visual control in order to identify the involved organs as the surgery progresses. Whenever initial adhesiolysis seems to progress easily, it should be continued; if, however, a particular movement does not seem to produce the desired effect, one should immediately abandon that approach and attempt a different one until the right cleavage plane is found. If the lack of success is due to the fibrous consistency of the adhesions, it is better not to pursue the intervention further, so as to avoid complications.

Adhesiolysis may produce hemorrhage that obscures the anatomical landmarks. Bleeding is usually the result of pursuing a "false route" and therefore serves to warn the operator that damage may have been done. The presence of blood adds to the risk of adhesion formation. From a practical point of view, whenever bleeding occurs, the surgeon should question whether it may not be better to stop the procedure at that point. The operator must also consider whether the blood should be completely evacuated and how hemostasis will be obtained. Rinsing the pelvis with warm physiologic solution is the first step in all cases. Very often this action alone will induce hemostasis. Subsequent reassessment of the site will then help in the decision as to whether to proceed or not. In the presence of persistent bleeding, bipolar coagulation (local bleeding) or use of vasopressin (diffuse bleeding) are useful. However, especially in the case of diffuse bleeding, spontaneous hemostasis will occur within minutes if one has the patience to wait. Occasionally, an intra-abdominal drain must be placed to monitor the bleeding further.

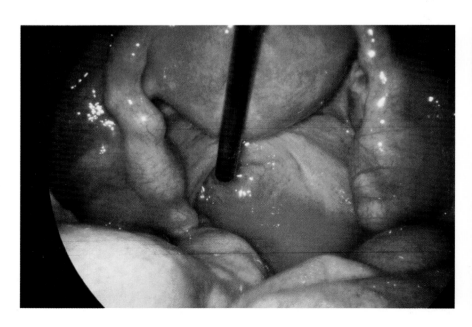

8.10 Sampling for bacteriology is followed by profuse rinsing of the pelvic cavity.

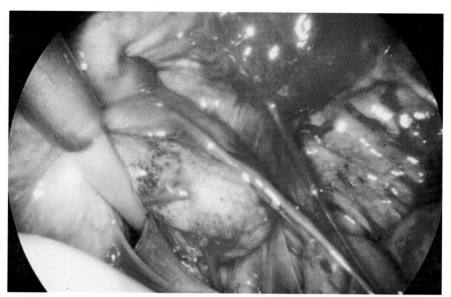

8.11*A* **and 8.11***B* Adhesiolysis is performed bluntly; scissors would be dangerous and less effective.

8.11*A*

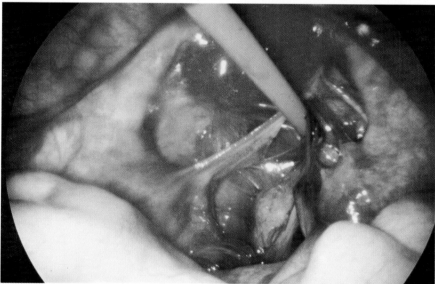

8.11*B*

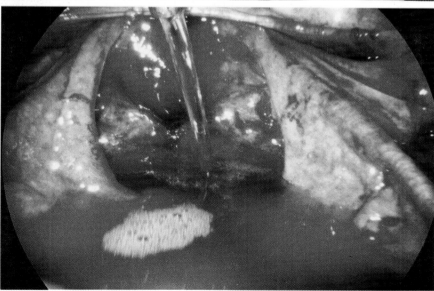

8.12 At completion of the adhesiolysis, irrigation with warm physiologic serum is used to obtain hemostasis.

Abscess drainage [26, 27, 34, 35, 38]

All abscesses must be drained; this is a basic rule in all surgery. The technique of drainage depends mainly on the location of the abscess.

Recent TOA

Adhesiolysis through rupture of adhesions and abscesses allows accurate diagnosis. Sometimes complete freeing up of the ovary and oviduct is not possible, especially when the bowel is heavily involved.

Recurrent TOA

Adhesiolysis in such a case is impossible. Indeed, puncture of only the most accessible areas is feasible. The failure rate of endoscopic treatment is therefore high, and it is questionable whether one should attempt it at all. Laparotomy may be the only choice.

Drainage of true pyosalpinx (Figs. 8.13 and 8.14)

Drainage calls for incision of the oviduct, ideally at the site of occlusion. Adhesiolysis is performed to mobilize the fallopian tube, and this is followed by incision of the occluded terminal end, as for salpingostomy. If mobilization of the tube seems unattainable, a longitudinal incision at the antimesenteric border is made as close to the fimbriated end as possible. The incision (using the monopolar needle) must be at least 1.5 cm long. Pus is aspirated and the lumen of the oviduct thoroughly rinsed for complete evacuation of the purulent material. These manipulations rarely cause bleeding. If oozing occurs at the surgical field, hemostasis can be obtained by injection of vasopressin in the same manner as for ectopic pregnancy.

The surgeon may encounter a number of difficulties: inability to mobilize the tube, an extremely thickened tubal wall, partitioning of the tubal lumen, etc. In such cases it is difficult to advocate a particular therapeutic approach; indeed, laparotomy may be required. Transverse incisions of the tubal wall are prohibited, because they can easily extend into complete transsection.

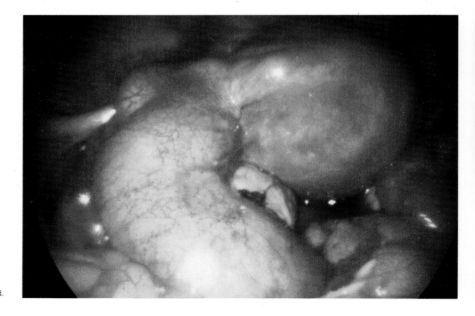

8.13 Large pyosalpinx of the left adnexa.

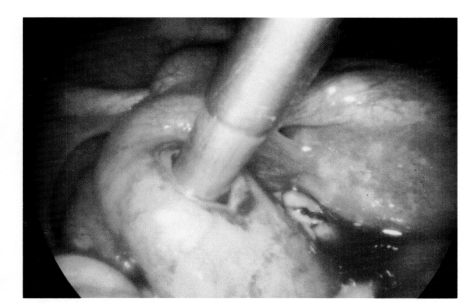

8.14A and 8.14B Drainage by incision of the pyosalpinx with the Triton (same patient as in 8.13).

8.14A

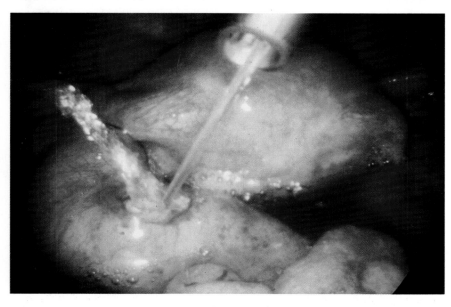

8.14B

Tubal abscess secondary to recent distal occlusion (Figs. 8.15 and 8.16)

Progressive, gentle, blunt dissection will extricate the fimbriated end from the tuboovarian complex. If occlusion occurred because of circumferential adhesion of the fimbriated end to surrounding structures, simple blunt dissection and mobilization will suffice to drain the pus. The rinsing probe is then introduced into the tube for lavage of its lumen.

If occlusion occurred by agglutination of the mucosal folds, adhesiolysis itself is not sufficient for drainage; opening of the distal end is required. A forceps is used to grasp the serosa of the ampulla and, with another, the velamentous adhesions among the mucosal folds are removed by simple traction. One should avoid grasping the mucosal folds themselves. Once the fimbrial os is identified, a blunt forceps is introduced gently in the closed position; the jaws of the forceps are then opened slightly and the instrument is slowly retrieved while in an open position. This will rupture the layers of fibrinous exudate. A thorough rinsing of the tubal lumen completes the procedure. This procedure is truly a fimbrioplasty; it is relatively easy and certainly bloodless.

Abscess of the pouch of Douglas

This problem is better approached by culdotomy rather than by drainage under endoscopic control.

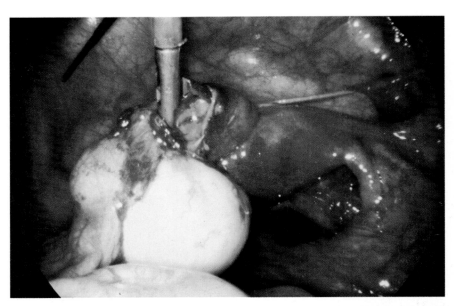

8.15 Opening of the agglutinated distal end of the tube allows drainage of the pyosalpinx.

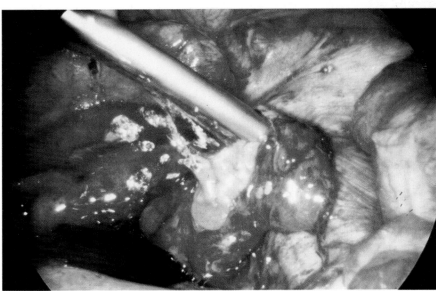

8.16 Drainage is followed by rinsing of the tubal lumen.

Peritoneal lavage (Fig. 8.17)

This is an absolutely essential part of the procedure. We use the Triton rinsing-aspiration device through a suprapubic puncture. The fluid is a warm physiologic solution (45° C) containing an antiseptic medium (Betadine). Rinsing should always be performed, even in the absence of abscess formation. The objectives are
   - Hemostasis by coagulation of the capillaries
   - Local antisepsis

Rinsing and evacuation of debris is a time-consuming process requiring specialized equipment that allows both rinsing and aspiration. During aspiration, the tip of the cannula is held just beneath the surface of the fluid to avoid aspiration of excessive amounts of CO_2. Plugging with appendices epiploicae or bowel can be avoided by holding a probe against the posterior aspect of the uterus or at the level of the ovarian ligament.

During the process of rinsing-evacuation, the Trendelenburg position is slowly reversed so as to permit evacuation of fluid that has accumulated above the pelvic brim.

At the end of this maneuver, fluid can be left inside as prophylaxis against adhesion formation. Physiologic solution is to be preferred over macromolecular solutions such as Dextran, which act as a growth medium for bacteria. An antiseptic can be added to the fluid. In our opinion, the most important role of the warm fluid left behind is hemostasis.

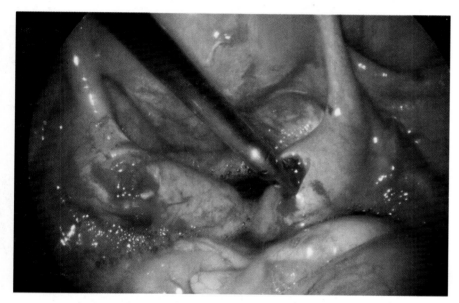

8.17*A* Incision of the antimesenteric border of the tube for drainage and rinsing of a bilateral pyosalpinx.

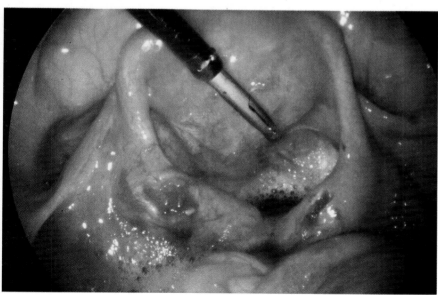

8.17*B* Situs at the end of the procedure (same patient as in 8.17).

Postoperative drainage

Postoperative drainage need not be performed in all cases. It is unnecessary if there was no abscess and if hemostasis was satisfactory. In all other cases, installation of a postoperative drain for 24 to 48 h is desirable to monitor recurrence of bleeding.

Antibiotics

Antibiotic treatment is initiated at the time of laparoscopy once sampling for bacteriology has been done. Numerous drug regimens have been advocated [11]. There is no clear advantage to any one of these schemes. Most of the data are based on clinical criteria—and their low degree of accuracy is well known. We recently performed a study based on objective criteria at second-look laparoscopy and have shown that a mefoxitin-doxycycline combination is less effective than ampicillin-penicillinase inhibitor-doxycycline [10, 35]. However, our objective is not to define the best antibiotic regimen. Broad-spectrum coverage is required and should be supplemented with 12 to 20 days of anti-*Chlamydia* treatment [39].

Postoperative care

Postoperative care consists of the usual surveillance of temperature, vital signs, abdominal distention, and intestinal function, especially if an abscess was drained. There should be no reason for reintervention during the first 72 h. Thereafter, if one considers treatment to have failed, laparoscopy should first be performed for confirmation, followed by laparotomy for extirpative surgery if required.

Results [34, 35]

Diagnostic value of second-look laparoscopy

Most studies on treatment of salpingitis base their data concerning incidence of healing on clinical observations, which we know to be unreliable. According to Burnham [11], one should look for
- Healing of the local infectious process
- Healing of the infection as a whole
- Fertility outcome

These criteria are indeed the most valuable, but they are difficult to obtain. We offer young patients with a desire for further fertility the option of a second-look laparoscopy for evaluation of sequelae of the infection [11, 34, 45]. At second-look laparoscopy, the following are assessed:
- Persistence of inflammatory reaction by cytology, biopsy of adhesions, and the overall aspect of the internal genital organs
- Tubal patency
- Extent of adhesions
- Necessity for tubal reconstructive surgery or medically assisted reproductive technology

Just how much time should elapse between the initial intervention and second-look laparoscopy has not been precisely determined. The interval should be long enough to allow complete healing but not so long as to delay diagnosis of persistent inflammation. Eight weeks seems to be a good interval.

Second-look laparoscopy is an objective means of assessing different treatment regimens. We have performed three such studies:
- Study 1: 34 patients—12 with exudative salpingitis, 11 with adhesion formation, and 11 with pelvic abscess [34]
- Study 2: 34 pyosalpinges (retrospective) [38]
- Study 3: 40 patients for randomized comparison of two antibiotic regimens [10]

The results are discussed below.

Persistence of inflammation

Inflammation persisted in 25 % of the patients in all three studies. Its presence is correlated only with the presence of *Chlamydia*. Whenever persistent infection is diagnosed, it should be treated with antibiotics, which probably limits long-term sequelae.

Tubal patency

Patency could be expected after treatment of acute salpingitis (91.1 %, study 1; 87 %, study 3) but came as a surprise after treatment of pelvic abscess (27.3 %, study 1; 32.3 %, study 2; 50 %, study 3). The outcome is better when the tubal occlusion was recent rather than recurrent. This amazing patency rate is the result of aggressive adhesiolysis. In the case of true pyosalpinx, patency depended on the type of drainage performed. When the tube was incised at the antimesenteric border, occlusion persisted. When salpingotomy was performed, 40 % of the oviducts remained patent (study 3). One of these patients later conceived and successfully carried a normal intrauterine pregnancy.

Adhesions

Adhesions afflict a high proportion of patients (73.5 %, study 1). Extent and type were related to the stage of the disease at the time of the initial diagnosis. Results in study 1 indicate that in 25 % of cases of acute salpingitis, in 90 % of cases in the agglutination stage, and in 100 % of cases with pelvic abscess, adhesions had formed. In all cases, complete adhesiolysis had been accomplished at the time of the initial procedure.

At first glance, one might conclude that adhesiolysis is of limited value. However, more detailed analysis shows that:
- Adhesions are less extensive at second-look laparoscopy.
- Initial adhesiolysis is absolutely necessary for accurate diagnosis and especially for drainage of abscesses, which is a condition sine qua non for complete healing.

One could therefore say that adhesiolysis at first laparoscopy is an integral part of diagnosis and treatment of the condition but does not constitute complete therapy.

Second-look laparoscopy is the ideal moment to complete reconstruction of the adnexae in at least three times out of four, when there are no remaining inflammatory lesions. (We obtained four intrauterine pregnancies in studies 1 and 3.)

Prognosis (fertility)

Prognosis depends on the stage of the disease at the time of diagnosis. In our first study, we evaluated the prognosis as being 91.7 %, 36.4 %, and 27.3 % in the exudative, agglutination, and pelvic abscess stages respectively. There seemed to be an indication for microsurgery in 8.3 %, 36.4 %, and 27.3 % and for in vitro fertilization in 8 %, 21.2 %, and 45.4 %, respectively.

During our third study, we were able to verify an impression we had earlier—that the prognosis depends on the status of the worst tube. For example, the rate of tubal patency of unilateral pyosalpinx combined with contralateral exudative salpingitis is the same as for bilateral pyosalpinx, namely 50 %.

Failure rate of laparoscopic treatment

Failure occurs only in the case of drainage of pyosalpinges. Delayed extirpative surgery occurs in 5 to 10 % [26, 34, 35, 38]–6.8 % in all our studies combined. This rate is lower than the failure rate of antibiotic treatment only (20 to 84 %) [5] and higher than that of radical surgery, which, however, induces irreversible sterility and has a high risk of bowel injury (2 to 8.5 %) [5].

What is the therapeutic role of second-look laparoscopy?

PID has three main consequences:
- Sterility
- Progressive deterioration of the pelvic organs
- High risk of recurrence

The formation of adhesions and hydrosalpinx is classical. This obviously leads to sterility, but complaints of infertility will be voiced by these women only several years later. Brosens and Vasquez [8] have demonstrated that the tubal epithelium of a hydrosalpinx undergoes progressive destruction; thus chances that reconstructive surgery will be successful diminish with the passage of time [28, 31]. Moreover, a hydrosalpinx is more prone to infection than is a patent tube. Reinfection of a hydrosalpinx automatically turns it into a pyosalpinx.

Second-look laparoscopy has several functions: to establish the cure, to assess the sequelae, and to correct the latter if necessary. Reconstructive surgery at second look encompasses adhesiolysis and/or salpingostomy. In fact, two patients whom we considered candidates for future microsurgery actually became pregnant following second-look treatment: one after extensive adhesiolysis and one after adhesiolysis and salpingostomy. Reconstructive surgery can be delayed [3, 9, 19]; however, we believe that it is imperative to perform reconstruction as soon after healing of PID as possible, even when there is no immediate desire for pregnancy. It is admittedly a new philosophical approach to treat the sequelae of PID in the absence of an immediate desire for pregnancy, but surgery is relatively easy soon after the infectious process has healed and becomes more difficult within only a few months.

Discussion

PID deserves more in-depth studies to fill in the many gaps in our knowledge about the disease. We would like to address some important questions.

Is laparoscopy mandatory for diagnosis of PID?

Laparoscopy remains the method par excellence for both morphologic and bacteriologic confirmation of the disease. The studies by Weström [42] have shown how difficult it is to diagnose PID on the basis of clinical signs only. All authors agree that:

– Laparoscopy is indicated for differential diagnosis with other pathology, such as ectopic pregnancy, torsion, endometriosis, appendicitis.

– Laparoscopy is indicated to confirm the presence of a pelvic abscess either at the start or the failure of antibiotic treatment.

We are convinced, like many others, that laparoscopy is an integral part of the evaluation of PID. One may argue that if all other investigations indicate the absence of pus collection, laparoscopy is of little value. An additional argument is that laparoscopy to examine sequelae following medical treatment is of greater value than laparoscopy for diagnosis and that the number of interventions should be limited to a minimum; therefore diagnostic laparoscopy should not be performed.

Elimination of the initial diagnostic endoscopy entails two questions: (1) is ultrasonography accurate in confirming the absence of pus collection? (2) How accurate is the diagnosis of PID without laparoscopy?

The answer to the first question remains unresolved. Our experience indicates that ultrasonography has limited accuracy [3, 4, 17, 37].

Paavonen answered the second question [33]. In 27 patients presenting clinical symptoms of PID, the following tests were performed: endometrial biopsy, peritoneal cytology, and laparoscopy. The endometrial biopsy showed a sensitivity of 89 %, a specificity of 67 %, and a false-negative rate of 22 %. With cytology, the values were, respectively, 75 %, 67 %, and 25 %. Therefore, these tests are not sufficiently accurate. Moreover, they tend to be aberrant in cases of early infection, which also have a poor clinical correlation.

Prevention remains a major objective [43]. It therefore seems illogical to us to deprive young patients, having a potential desire for fertility, of the benefits of diagnostic laparoscopy. Medical treatment without prior laparoscopy is acceptable only in patients bearing obvious clinical signs, having an absence of indications for present pyosalpinx, and having no further desire for fertility. This is particularly true in patients who have had previous episodes of PID. On the other hand, when there is only slight clinical suspicion and laparoscopy seems too invasive for confirmation of the diagnosis, antibiotic treatment is not the appropriate treatment either. Rather, expectant management for 2 to 4 days is more appropriate. When signs do not abate, laparoscopy should be performed. Indeed, minimal treatment increases the risk for incomplete treatment, leading to a greater risk for sequelae.

Is there still an indication for extirpative surgery in the presence of pyosalpinx?

Exeresis is still the standard treatment, unfortunately. It should be abandoned in favor of laparoscopic drainage. There remain some indications for the removal of affected organs, especially in the older patients having no desire for further fertility and in patients who have already had several recurrences. A difficult dilemma is the presence of a pyosalpinx with a normal-appearing contralateral tube. Drainage may contaminate the healthy tube and cause adhesions. It seems acceptable to remove the affected tube in such a case [10, 14, 26, 34, 37], although no study supports this approach. In all other cases, the preferred treatment is laparoscopic drainage.

When is a second-look laparoscopy indicated?

This question encompasses two factors: patient selection and time interval. The objective of the second look is to detect persistent inflammation, evaluate the prognosis, treat the sequelae, and devise a proper therapeutic plan.

Laparoscopy is the method of choice to establish arrest of the inflammatory process [11, 34, 45].

– Clinical evaluation is based mainly on pain symptoms, which are difficult to interpret except in acute salpingitis.

– Biochemical tests are of value only to follow the evolution of a known infection. CBC and ESR can be quite normal in the presence of progressive disease [35].

– Persistence of inflammatory reaction is independent of the extent of the disease at diagnosis but is related to the infectious agent: *Chlamydia* infections [10] more often lead to chronic disease.

Sequelae are related to the extent of the disease at diagnosis (e.g., in the presence of acute salpingitis, sequelae are rather uncommon) [34].

We defend the attitude that second-look laparoscopy should be offered to those patients with a desire for future fertility except if one is dealing with acute salpingitis without *Chlamydia*, which leads only rarely (<10%) to sequelae.

The ideal interval is difficult to choose. Two months is an ideal compromise between overrating persistent infection and late diagnosis of subclinical chronic infection. A longer latency period could be chosen in case of *Chlamydia* infection treated with tetracycline for a long period of time.

The main objective of second-look laparoscopy is diagnosis and treatment of sequelae. Thus, the second look should be performed when one is convinced that the infectious process has ceased. This brings up the question whether other tests can be helpful in diagnosing resolution of the infection. We have no answer to this question, which requires prospective studies. One may state that if such tests were available, second-look laparoscopy would not be necessary in cases of acute salpingitis that healed well. In all other cases, the procedure would be done after it had been established that the infection was cured except if the course of the disease indicated incorrect initial diagnosis or unsatisfactory initial endosurgical treatment.

Second-look laparoscopy is certainly a must for evaluation of treatment modalities, either surgical or medical [10, 35]. Evaluation of sequelae can serve as a scientifically acceptable marker of success in lieu of long-term fecundity rates, which are difficult to handle in a patient population with, a priori, diverging desires for further fertility.

There are many aspects deserving further evaluation: the healing process of various tissues, the pathophysiology of changes in peritoneal cytology, biochemical markers for pelvic infections and their correlation with future fertility, etc.

References

1. Abeille J.P., Tomikowski G., Legros R., « Dosages péritonéaux per-cœlioscopiques et sériques de l'orosomucoïde et d'autres marqueurs de l'inflammation dans l'étude des processus inflammatoires pelviens », *Gynécol.*, 1983; 34 : 519-525.
2. Adhesion Study Group, « Reduction of post-operative pelvic adhesions with intraperitoneal 32 % dextran: a prospective, randomized clinical trial », *Fertil. Steril.*, 1983; 40 : 612-619.
3. Berlend L.L., Lawson T.L., Foley W.D., Albanelli J.N., « Ultrasound evaluation of pelvic infections », *Radiol. Clin. North Am.*, 1982; 20 : 367-382.
4. Bessis R., « Infection pelvienne et échographie », *Contrac. Fertil. Sexual.*, 1984; suppl. 12 : 329-336.
5. Bieluch W.M., Tally F.P., « Pathophysiology of abscess formation », *Clin. Obstet. Gynecol.*, 1983; 10 : 93-103.
6. Blum F., Pathier D., Treisser A., Faguer C., Barrat J., « Infections génitales hautes aiguës. 1. Etude clinique et apport de la cœlioscopie », *J. Gynecol. Obstet. Biol. Reprod.*, 1979; 8 : 711-721.
7. Blum F., Tessier F., Pathier D., Treisser A., Faguer C., Barrat J., « Infections génitales hautes aiguës. 2. Etude bactériologique et conséquences thérapeutiques », *J. Gynecol. Obstet. Biol. Reprod.*, 1980; 9 : 229-242.
8. Brosens I., Boeckx W., Vasquez G., Winston R., « Selection des candidates pour la plastie tubaire »; in: Oviducte et fertilité, Masson, Paris, 1979, p. 367.
9. Bruhat M.A., Mage G., Manhes H., Soualhat C., Ropert J.F., Pouly J.L., « Laparoscopic procedures to promote fertility: ovariolysis and salpingolysis; results of 93 selected cases », *Acta Eur. Fertil.*, 1983; 14 : 113-116.
10. Bruhat M.A., Pouly J.L., Mage G., Le Bouedec G., « Treatment of acute salpingitis with sulbactam/ampicillin. Comparison with cefoxitin », *Drugs*, 1986; 31 (suppl. 2), 7-10.
11. Brunham R., « Therapy of acute pelvic inflammatory disease: a critique of recent treatment trials », *Am. J. Obstet. Gynecol.*, 1984; 148 : 235-240.
12. Catalan F., Khoury B., Ouizman E., « Nouvelles méthodes de diagnostic des infections à *Chlamydia* », *Rev. Fr. Gynecol. Obstet.*, 1984; 79 : 617-623.
13. De Brux J., Mintz M., « Exploration cyto-histopathologique du péritoine pelvien »; in: Le tissu cellulaire pelvien, Masson, Paris, 1973, pp. 133-156.
14. Dorez F., Cavaille F., Sureau C., « Hypothèses relatives aux variations de mobilité des spermatozoïdes dans le liquide péritonéal », *J. Gynecol. Obstet. Biol. Reprod.*, 1985; 14 : 955-958.
15. Eschenbach D., Buchanan T.R., Pollock H.M., « Polymicrobial etiology of acute inflammatory disease », *N. Engl. J. Med.*, 1975, 293 : 166-171.
16. Forrest J., Buckley Ch., Fox H., « Pelvic endometriosis and tubal inflammatory disease », *Int. J. Gynecol. Path.*, 1984; 3 : 343-347.
17. Golde S.H., « Unilateral tubo-ovarian abscess: a distinct entity », *Am. J. Obstet. Gynecol.*, 1977; 127 : 807-810.
18. Golditch I.M., Huston J.E., « Serious pelvic infections associated with intra-uterine contraceptive device », *Int. J. Fertil.*, 1973; 18 : 156-160.
19. Gomel V., « Salpingo-ovariolysis by laparoscopy in infertility », *Fertil. Steril.*, 1983; 40 : 607-611.
20. Hager W.D., « Follow-up of patients with tubo-ovarian abscess in association with salpingitis », *Obstet. Gynecol.*, 1983; 61 : 680-684.
21. Henri-Suchet, J., Gayraud M., « Annexites non tuberculeuses, valeur de la cœlioscopie dans le diagnostic, le traitement et l'évaluation d'un pronostic tubaire »; in: Infection et fertilité, Masson, Paris, 1977, p. 199.
22. Henri-Suchet J., Paris F.X., Catalan F., « Place de *Chlamydia trachomatis* dans l'étiologie des salpingites aiguës », *Presse Méd.*, 1983; 12 : 2869-2872.
23. Henri-Suchet J., Goldstein F., Acar J., « Etude bactériologique des prélèvements cœlioscopiques dans les annexites aiguës », *J. Gynecol. Obstet. Biol. Reprod.*, 1980; 9 : 341-346.
24. Henri-Suchet J., Catalan F., Loffredo V., « Etude microbiologique des prélèvements cœlioscopiques dans les annexites et les stérilités tubaires », *J. Gynecol. Obstet. Biol. Reprod.*, 1980; 9 : 445-453.
25. Henri-Suchet J., « Salpingites aiguës et silencieuses. Aspect actuel », *Contrac. Fertil Sexual.*, 1984; suppl. 12 : 229-234.
26. Henri-Suchet J., Soler A., Loffredo V., « Laparoscopic treatment of tubo-ovarian abscesses », *Int. J. Reprod. Med.*, 1984; 29 : 579-582.
27. Henri-Suchet J., Chahine N., Loffredo V., « Adhésiolyse cœlioscopique et traitement des abcès pelviens au cours des salpingites aiguës (78 cas) », *Gynécologie*, 1981; 24 : 419-424.
28. Henri-Suchet J., « Endoscopie tubaire: premiers résultats », *Gynécologie*, 1981; 23 : 293-298.
29. Jacobson L., « Differential diagnosis of acute pelvic inflammatory diseases », *Am. J. Obstet. Gynecol.*, 1980; 136 : 1006-1011.
30. Mac-Gowan L., Bunnag B., « A morphological classification of peritoneal fluid cytology in women », *Int. J. Gynecol. Obstet.*, 1973; 11 : 173-180.

31. Mage G., Pouly J.L., Bouquet de Jolinière J., Chabrand S., Bruhat M.A., « Obstructions tubaires distales: microchirurgie ou fécondation *in vitro* », *J. Gynecol. Obstet. Biol. Reprod.*, 1984; 13 : 933-937.
32. Monif G.R., « Clinical staging of acute bacterial salpingitis and its therapeutic ramifications », *Am. J. Obstet. Gynecol.*, 1982; 142 : 489-495.
33. Paavonen J., Aine R., Teisala K., Heinonen P., Punnonen R., « Comparison of endometrial biopsy and peritoneal fluid cytologic testing with laparoscopy in the diagnosis of acute pelvic inflammatory disease », *Am. J. Obstet. Gynecol.*, 1985; 151 : 645-650.
34. Pouly J.L., Mage G., Dupre B., Canis M., Bruhat M.A., « Cœlioscopie de contrôle précoce après salpingite », *J. Gynecol. Obstet. Biol. Reprod.*, 1985; 14 : 989-996.
35. Pouly J.L., Le Bouedec G., Mage G., Bruhat M.A., « Cœlioscopie de contrôle précoce après salpingite: étude randomisée comparative sulbactam-ampicilline contre céfoxitine », (à paraître).
36. Schmidt C.L., Demopoulos R.I., Weiss G., « Infected endometriotic cysts: clinical characterization and pathogenesis », *Fertil. Steril.*, 1981; 36 : 27-33.
37. Spirtos N.J., Bernstine R.L., Crawford W.L., « Sonography in acute pelvic inflammatory diseases », *J. Reprod. Med.*, 1982; 27 : 312-320.
38. Stener V., « Traitement cœlioscopique des pyosalpinx », Thèse de Médecine, Faculté de Médecine de Clermont-Ferrand, 1986.
39. Sweet R.L., « Chlamydial salpingitis and infertility », *Fertil. Steril.*, 1982; 38 : 62-68.
40. Sweet R.L., Draper D.L., et al., « Microbiology and pathogenesis of acute salpingitis as determined by laparoscopy. What is the appropriate site to sample », *Am. J. Obstet. Gynecol.*, 1980; 131 : 885-889.
41. Wang S.G., Eschenbach D.A., Holmes K.K., Wager G., Crayston J.T., « *Chlamydia trachomatis* infection in Fitz-Hugh-Curtis syndrome », *Am. J. Obstet. Gynecol.*, 1980; 131 : 1034-1038.
42. Weström L., « Effect of pelvic inflammatory disease on fertility », *Am. J. Obstet. Gynecol.*, 1975; 121 : 707-713.
43. Weström L., « Epidémiologie des salpingites et leurs conséquence », *Contrac. Fertil. Sexual.*, 1984; suppl. 12 : 235-241.
44. Wheeler J.E., « Pathology of the fallopian tube »; in: Pathology of the female genital tract », Ed. by Blaumstein A., 2nd, édit., 1982; 397-400.
45. Wolner-Hanssen P., Weström L., « Second look laparoscopy after acute salpingitis », *Obstet. Gynecol.*, 1983; 61 : 702-704.

9
Adhesions

Adhesions are bridges of newly formed fibrous tissue connecting two organs that are normally separated. Their incidence is relatively high in patients presenting with infertility or chronic pelvic pain [8, 40]. Whatever the etiology of the adhesions, definitive diagnosis is possible only by laparoscopy even if sequestration of the dye at hysterosalpingography is highly suggestive of their presence, as in the case of known previous surgery or pelvic inflammatory disease (PID). The great potential of the endosurgical approach warrants discussion in this separate chapter.

Pathophysiology

Etiology

Three major processes cause peritoneal lesions that lead to adhesion formation:
- PID
- Surgical trauma
- Endometriosis

PID

PID is the main culprit in adhesion formation. The primary cause is ascending infection, but secondary spread from another site, as from an infected appendix, may occur. Absence of risk factors in the patient's history and scant symptomatology do not exclude the presence of PID, for the work by Jacobson and Weström [33] has demonstrated a silent course of the disease in 15 % of cases.

Surgical trauma

Any laparotomy may cause adhesion formation, but the incidence is higher in case of [13, 17]:
- Ovarian cystectomy
- Ovarian wedge-resection, which causes adhesion formation in all cases, according to Buttram and Vaquero [10]
- Myomectomy and uteroplasty
- Extrauterine pregnancy
- Oophorectomy and salpingectomy
- Appendectomy

Gordji and Palmer found that 40 % of women presenting with pelvic adhesions had undergone appendectomy, whereas the incidence of appendectomy in the general population is only 10 % [26].

Several factors play a role in the pathogenesis of adhesion formation:
- Presence of blood associated with dryness or trauma of the peritoneal surface
- Foreign material—such as talc, gauze, etc.—because of the resulting inflammatory reaction
- Ischemia of the tissue, which should be minimized through avoidance of tight peritoneal sutures [3]

All these factors have led to the principles of tubal microsurgery: minimal tissue trauma, copious irrigation with heparinized Ringer's lactate at body temperature, rinsing of surgical gloves, minimal use of gauze, meticulous hemostasis, careful peritonealization with sutures and free peritoneal grafts, and reduced surgical time [28].

Endometriosis

Endometriosis is the causative agent in 15 % of cases and may be difficult to recognize, especially when the implants are located on the lateral aspect of the ovarian surface. Quite often, it is only after mobilization of the ovary that the presence of endometriotic implants or a small endometrioma becomes clear, thereby excluding an infectious etiology. A similar problem in differential diagnosis occurs in cul-de-sac obliteration. However, differentiation is vital in view of initiating appropriate therapy.

Mechanisms of infertility

Most often, adhesions are associated with distal tubal pathology, which in itself explains infertility. This is particularly true following salpingitis. Apparently normal tubal morphology is, however, not uncommon, especially following pelvic surgery, appendectomy, or peritonitis. Infertility is then caused by an altered anatomic relationship between tube and ovary, interfering with ovum pickup and, in particular, reducing tubal motility [4]. To affect fertility, the adhesions must be relatively extensive and bilateral (or unilateral when only a single adnexa is present). The occurrence of an intrauterine pregnancy in a patient with relatively normal-appearing oviducts less than 12 months following adhesiolysis testifies to the role of mechanical obstruction by adhesions in infertility.

There are, however, two more mechanisms through which infertility is caused by adhesions:

– Periovarian adhesions may lead to ovarian dysfunction, as was suggested several years ago by Abeille [1]. In the meantime, multiple studies in IVF centers have supported this finding.

– Association with ovarian or peritoneal endometriosis, which by itself could explain failure to conceive.

Classification of adhesions

Adhesions present various morphologies, necessitating a classification to facilitate both description and evaluation of the prognosis of the condition. Three aspects are of primary importance.

Morphology

Palmer [36] described three different types of adhesions (Figs. 9.1 through 9.4):

– *Type A —filmy:* These adhesions are thin, avascular, and form veil-like sheets between organs or cocoons around them.

– *Type B —vascular:* These adhesions are similar to type A but are vascular.

– *Type C —dense:* These adhesions result in tight, thick connective bridges between organs.

This classification, established several years ago, does not take into account the various morphokinetic stages of healing and scar formation. We hypothesize nowadays that the adhesions labeled type B are actually an intermediary state and are in the process of evolving toward either type A or type C. This theory, however, still needs to be proved.

The AFS classification (1985) for endometriosis considers only two classes of adhesions: filmy and dense.

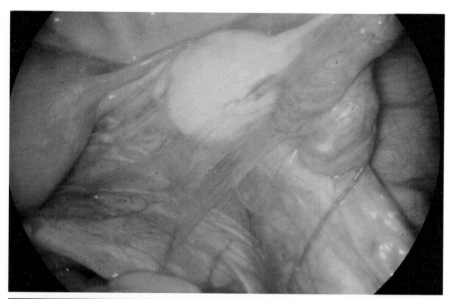

The three main types of adhesions, as described by Raoul Palmer:

9.1 Type A: Filmy adhesion.

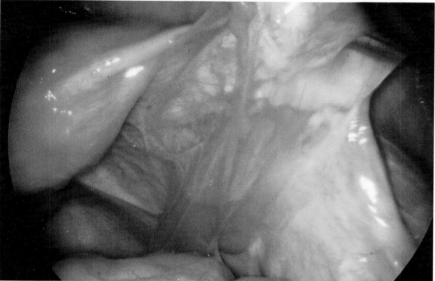

9.2 Type B: Vascular adhesion.

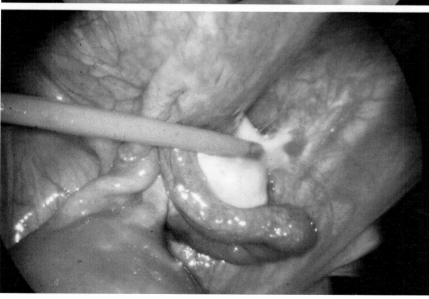

9.3 Type C: Dense adhesion.

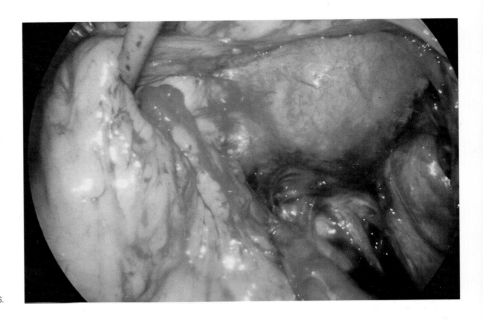

9.4 Omental adhesions.

Extent of adhesions

The extent of adhesions must be determined. This requires complete exploration of the pelvis. The simplest method is to evaluate the proportion of the
organ that is involved in adhesions, particularly the proportion of the oviduct
and the ovary. Numerous classifications have been proposed [7, 11, 30, 31, 34,
36, 46].

Our data have taken into account the type and extent of the adhesion and
have enabled us to establish an adhesion score for each adnexa, so that we can
evaluate the extent of disease (Table 9.1). We distinguish three stages (mild,
moderate, and severe), and these are correlated with fertility outcome after
adhesiolysis or distal tubal surgery [37].

TABLE 9.1   **Classification of adhesions according to the authors**[a]

For each adnexa	type A: filmy, avascular type B: dense or vascular type C: obliteration			
			Surface		
Ovary	Absence	1/4	2/4	3/4	4/4
A	0	1	1	1	1
B	0	2	4	6	10
C	0	5	10	15	20
Isthmus tubae	Absence	1/3 (attached)	2/3 (encapsulated)	3/3 (fixed)
A	0	1	1	1
B	0	1	3	6
C	0	3	5	10
Ampulla tubae	Absence	1/3 (attached)	2/3 (encapsulated)	3/3 (fixed)
A	0	1	1	1
B	0	2	4	6
C	0	5	10	15

[a]Four stages: absence, score = 0; mild, 1–9; moderate, 10–19; severe, ≥20.

It is also possible to utilize the classification proposed by the American Fertility Society in 1985, which is somewhat simpler (Table 9.2). In our experience, however, the use of either of these two classifications does not modify the final staging of the disease and therefore of the prognosis.

TABLE 9.2 **AFS classification of pelvic adhesions**[a]

Organ	Type	Surface involved		
		1/3	2/3	3/3
Ovaries	Filmy	1	2	4
	Dense	4	8	16
Ampulla tubae	Filmy	1	2	4
	Dense	4	8	16

[a]Absence, 0; mild, 1–10; moderate, 11–16; severe, >16.

Evolution of adhesions

Adhesions resulting from salpingectomy or appendectomy are stable, because they represent scar tissue. Conversely, adhesions observed during the healing phase of a salpingitis are in the process of evolving. Between these two extremes, there are a number of instances in which adhesions are potentially progressive, but this is not evident either clinically or macroscopically. It is especially important that such cases be diagnosed before microsurgical or endosurgical interventions are undertaken, because—without prior medical treatment—recurrence and even worsening of the condition will almost certainly ensue.

Classically, progressive adhesions have an edematous and vascular appearance. However, in practice, macroscopic evaluation is unreliable and cannot be considered definitive. The potential of adhesions to be progressive must be evaluated by using objective criteria, such as histologic examination and peritoneal cytology [6, 14, 15, 35]. Also, it is of utmost importance, prior to beginning any endoscopic procedure in the presence of adhesions, to sample the peritoneal fluid prior to surgery, so as to avoid contamination with sanguinous exudate. Biopsy of the adhesions is also recommended. If these tests reveal an ongoing inflammatory process, long-term postoperative medical treatment with antibiotics and anti-inflammatory agents must be undertaken to increase the likelihood of success.

This is very often neglected and may explain quite a number of failures of otherwise technically perfect endosurgical procedures.

Operative techniques

Description of the operative technique is difficult, because it varies according to the instruments used and the type and location of the adhesions. However, there are general principles that must be observed (Figs. 9.5 to 9.18).

General principles

Endosurgical adhesiolysis can be performed with either forceps and scissors or CO_2 laser.

The first technique is the simplest and least expensive. The laser, in our opinion, offers only a modest improvement in adhesiolysis—specifically, when dealing with adhesions located in particular sites and resulting from particular etiologies.

For more details on instrumentation, please refer to Chapter 2.

9.5–9.9 An example of adhesiolysis: two retro-pubic trocars are necessary. Note that the operator proceeds from "easy" to "difficult" (Figs. 9.6 and 9.7) and from medial to lateral. Peritoneal lavage completes the intervention, leaving 100 to 200 mL of warm physiologic solution intraperitoneally.

9.5

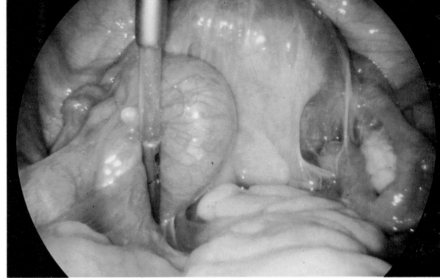

9.6

9.7

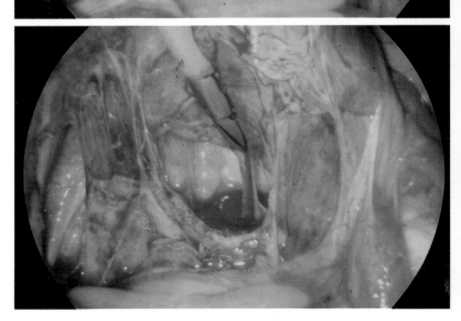

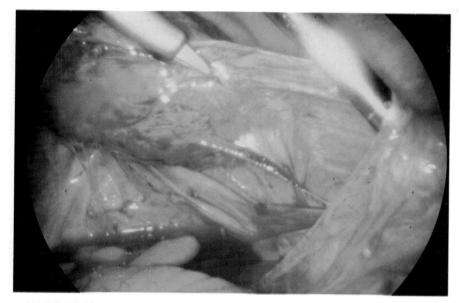

9.8

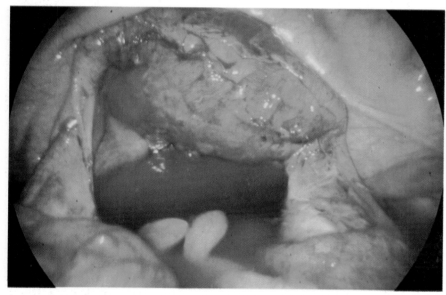

9.9

All adhesiolysis, but especially extensive adhesiolysis, calls for the use of two or three suprapubic trocars.

The degree of difficulty depends on the type of adhesion. Dissection of type A adhesions is easy, but type B adhesions call for more rigorous technique because of their vascular character. Type C adhesions are especially difficult to treat and, in fact, endosurgical treatment should be attempted only if they involve organs such as the uterus and ovary or if their extent is limited.

Adhesions should be sectioned or resected only after they have been put under tension. The adhesion must be meticulously defined and put under tension, using a probe or atraumatic forceps, then sectioned at its two extremities, paying attention to the visceral peritoneum of the involved organs. Section and resection are always preferable to careless rupture with a probe. The latter, in fact, produces areas of deperitonealization, which may cause the recurrence of adhesions. When traction on the adhesion is difficult, due either to the site of the adhesion (tubo-ovarian adhesion) or to its particular type (type C), one must perform very gentle dissection with a sharp scissors. This initial dissection usually allows the introduction of an atraumatic forceps, which then, secondarily, permits the adhesion to be put under tension by separation of its blades. This maneuver is extremely difficult and sometimes induces hemorrhage. In such a case, one must abandon the dissection, because it is obviously counterproductive to perform adhesiolysis and, by the procedure itself, create large zones of deperitonealization (which will then cause recurrences that may be more severe than the initial lesions). However, when apparently extensive adhesions are encountered, one should not immediately assume that the task is insurmountable. Once the initial plane is incised, the rest of the intervention may be surprisingly easy.

One should proceed from the simple to the more complex. It is therefore preferable to start adhesiolysis by sectioning filmy adhesions, so as to get a better grip on the denser areas. In general, an intervention proceeds from midline toward side wall, the adhesions blocking access to the cul-de-sac being transected first, and then proceeding toward the adnexa. However, in certain cases, one should make exceptions to the rule. For instance, the difficulty of tubo-ovarian adhesiolysis is related to the mobility of the two organs. Therefore, if the ovary is densely adherent to the posterior aspect of the broad ligament, one should leave it untouched until after salpingolysis has been performed, because salpingolysis will be facilitated by fixation of the ovary in its fossa.

Endosurgical adhesiolysis must follow the rules of microsurgery. The endoscope must be brought close enough to the operative field to obtain the magnification necessary for surgical precision. If the adhesiolysis is lengthy, one should take an overview of the pelvis from time to time so as to reestablish, in the surgeon's mind, the anatomic relationship of the various organs, and facilitate a decision on the next step to be taken in the procedure.

Hemostasis must be immediate and meticulous if the bleeding involves an artery or a vein. Bipolar coagulation is preferable to monopolar (dangerous) and thermocoagulation (somewhat imprecise). Hemostasis of capillary bleeding is obtained by continuously rinsing with physiologic solution. It is very often necessary, during adhesiolysis, to repeat peritoneal lavage several times, so as to avoid imprecise surgical manipulations on tissue covered by blood clots. Preventive use of vasopressin is, in many cases, an elegant alternative to these problems.

At the end of adhesiolysis, peritoneal lavage with warm saline should be routine and is mandatory. In this way, small clots are evacuated and one can also assess whether hemostasis is complete. If the ovarian cortex is bleeding, it is preferable to obtain hemostasis with bipolar coagulation or by infiltration of the infundibulopelvic ligament or ovarian ligament with vasopressin. Bleeding points on the posterior aspect of the uterus are equally accessible to hemostasis with electrocautery. However, bleeding originating from the posterior aspect of the broad ligament is difficult and sometimes even dangerous to deal with; we would prefer, in these cases, to tolerate a certain amount of oozing, which can be monitored by intraperitoneal drainage without suction for 24 to 48 h.

At the end of intervention, various solutions have been instilled intraperitoneally to avoid adhesions. None of them have proved really efficacious except perhaps for Dextran 70. However, this product has disadvantages that have led us to abandon its use. We leave only 100 to 200 mL of physiologic saline or Ringer's lactate intraperitoneally. Perhaps, at some time in the future, biologic glue will occupy an important place in the prevention of the recurrence of adhesions in areas of adhesiolysis. Currently, there are no data to support this statement, but preliminary trials are encouraging.

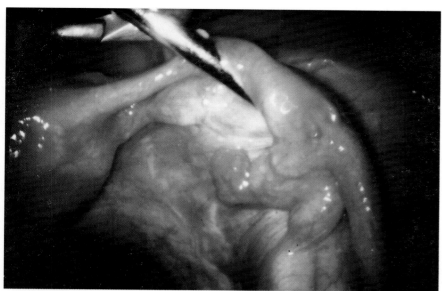

9.10–9.18 Adhesiolysis of right adnexa in a patient with infertility.

9.10 Initial situs: tubo-ovarian adhesions; ovary encased in broad ligament; ampulla tubae adherent to cranial pole of the ovary and round ligament.

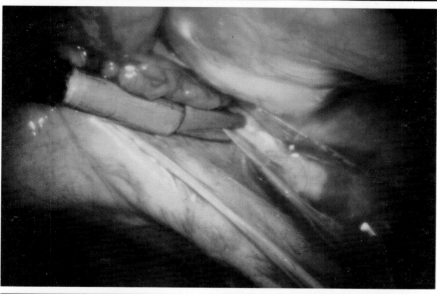

9.11 Lysis of distal end of the tube from the posterior leaf of the broad ligament.

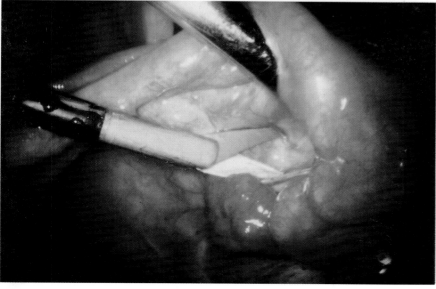

9.12 Initial ovariolysis, uncovering the ovarian surface.

9.13–9.15 Lysis of ampulla tubae from cranial pole of ovary. Note the blunt dissection that always precedes section. The ovary is still trapped in the broad ligament, which facilitates the dissection.

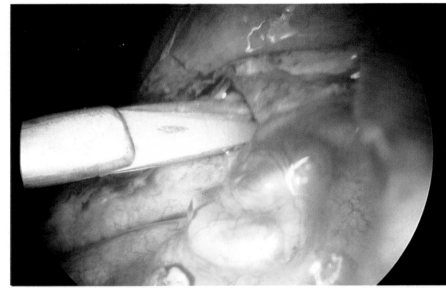

9.13

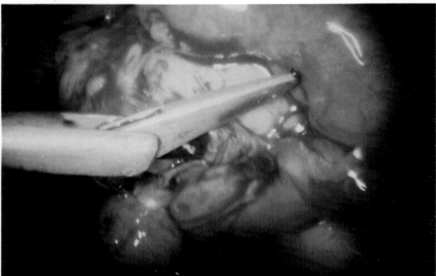

9.14

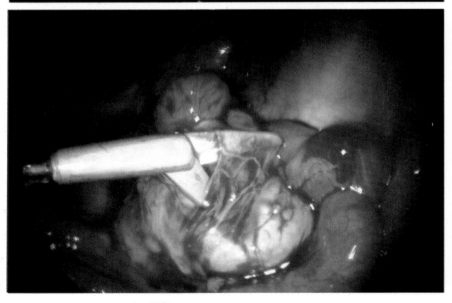

9.15

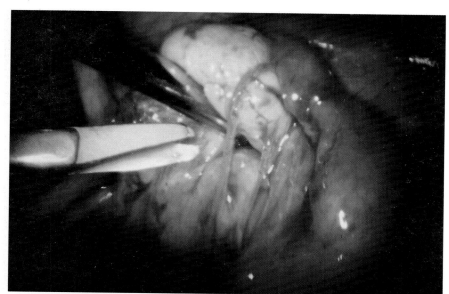

9.16–9.17 Lysis of ovary from broad ligament.

9.16

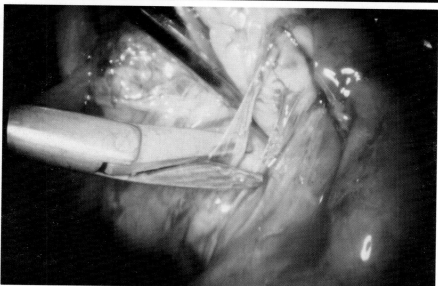

9.17

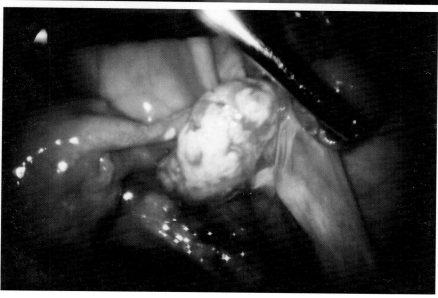

9.18 Final situs: the ovary and tube are free of adhesions (the distal tubal end is masked by the trocar sleeve). The intervention is completed by peritoneal lavage and chromopertubation with methylene blue.

Postoperative care

The duration of hospitalization is between 24 and 72 h, according to the extent of the adhesiolysis and the degree of hemostasis. Recovery of bowel function occurs within 24 h. Postoperative peritoneal drainage should be brief—24 to 48 h. This is sufficient to detect postoperative hemorrhage, which may necessitate a second endoscopy or other surgical intervention. In practice, the appearance is more important than the quantity in determining when to remove the drain:

— Within the first 6 h, it is not uncommon for the drain to yield 400 to 500 mL of serosanginous fluid, which corresponds, for the most part, to the remains of the rinsing fluid used during the intervention.

— Thereafter, peritoneal drainage usually does not stop completely and removal of the drain is permissible if only 100 to 150 mL of slightly blood-tinged fluid is obtained. Reintervention is justified only if the drain yields frankly bloody fluid 48 to 72 h after the first intervention.

The nursing staff needs to be educated in how to monitor the drains. Because no suction is involved, the drains operate on the principle of communicating vessels. Sometimes (in fact, frequently), it happens that, when the patient stands up or when the flask is held above the level of the patient's abdomen, the drainage stops. Therefore, to reestablish the drainage, one should either ask the patient to cough or gently push on her abdomen.

Minor intestinal complaints are frequently observed during the first postoperative week. Rarely, one may be confronted with more severe symptoms that could lead to the diagnosis of occlusion. Three different etiologic origins should be considered:

— Reflex ileus secondary to instillation of Dextran
— Fast recurrence of adhesions, especially if they involve the bowel
— Persistence of a low-rate hemorrhage that forms a hematocele

The latter can easily be diagnosed with physical examination and ultrasonography. These difficult situations are rather rare, but they may necessitate reintervention, which might be possible endosurgically for an experienced surgeon. An intestinal perforation which goes unnoticed during the surgical procedure generally leads rather rapidly to a dramatic clinical picture, diagnosable on the evening of or the day following an endosurgical procedure.

Technique of adhesiolysis according to site of adhesions

The purpose of this section is to discuss the details appropriate to each particular site.

Adhesions between the tube and the parietal peritoneum

The adhesion can be put under tension by either grasping the tube and displacing it medially or introducing a forceps between the tube and side wall at the level of or beneath the infundibulopelvic ligament.

One must distinguish between two different situations related to the type of adhesion:

— If one is confronted with filmy adhesions, sectioning is easy, but it must be done with care to avoid injuring the infundibulopelvic ligament or the ureter.

— If one is dealing with extremely dense adhesions (type C), adhesiolysis may be difficult; sometimes a cleavage plane is created lateral to the ovary, which may have severe consequences. Moreover, the outcome of adhesiolysis in these cases is poor, in view of the high rate of recurrence. Adhesiolysis using microsurgical techniques at laparotomy is therefore preferable, because satisfactory reperitonealization can be obtained either by suturing or by free peritoneal grafts. Finally, in less experienced hands, endosurgical interventions might result in irreversible damage to the tube.

Tubo-ovarian adhesions (Figs. 9.19 and 9.20)

The importance of tubo-ovarian mobility is quite well known. The difficulty in adhesiolysis results from the extreme mobility of those two organs.

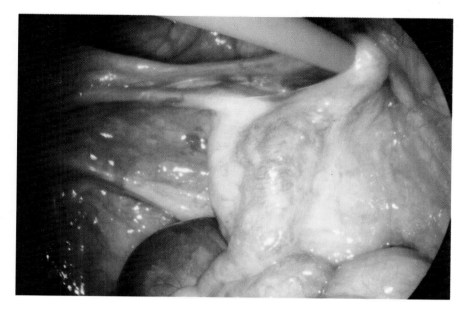

9.19 Adhesions of type A and type C between ampulla tubae and ovary. The probe between tube and ovary puts the adhesions under tension for easier lysis.

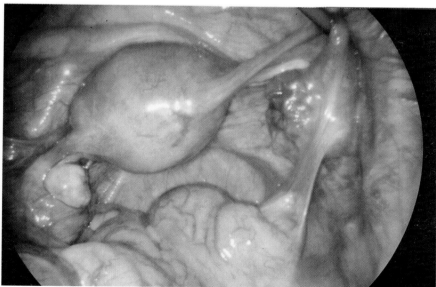

9.20 Vascular adhesion between oviduct and bowel. The probe elevates the oviduct for stretching the adhesion, which is then cut alongside the tube. Without mobilization of the tube, neither diagnosis nor section of this adhesion would have been possible.

Filmy adhesions

Grasping the tube with atraumatic forceps and displacing it upward usually yields sufficient traction. Scissors can then be inserted into the mesenteric recess created by the mesosalpinx. Progressively opening the scissors causes the adhesions to rupture into isolated strands, which can then be cut. Sectioning should be done slowly and progressively, a couple of millimeters at a time, taking care to remain close to the ovarian surface. It is common to encounter successive layers of adhesions. The difficulty here is to recognize the mesosalpinx and not to incise it. Therefore gentle, blunt dissection with the scissors should always precede sectioning. This type of adhesiolysis should always be performed from the midline toward the side wall. It is extremely important to explore the entire course of the tube carefully, so as to detect adhesions that can easily be overlooked, especially at the level of the proximal portion of the isthmus.

At the level of the infundibulum, the technique is similar, but the procedure must be very carefully carried out, with even more attention paid to blunt dissection. This is to avoid involuntary incision of the mesosalpinx at the level of the terminal artery, which vascularizes the infundibulum. Section of this vessel is a serious complication, because hemostasis will require excessive application of bipolar electrical current, with subsequent anatomic and functional impairment of the tube. Injection of vasopressin is preferable for hemostasis of lesions of the mesosalpinx.

Dense adhesions

The approach here is somewhat different. In the first step, the ovarian ligament is grasped to rotate the ovary upward, thereby presenting the dense adhesion to the operator. An atraumatic forceps with smooth edges will initiate the dissection of the cleavage plane between the ovary and the tube. When blunt dissection has proceeded over 1 to 2 cm by progressively introducing the blunt forceps parallel to the course of the mesosalpinx, the forceps is held open to produce tension on the dense adhesion which, in turn, is sectioned with scissors. This approach is repeated until the entire tube is freed.

Dense adhesions connecting the infundibulum and the ovary are particularly difficult to approach endosurgically. As much as possible, this adhesiolysis should be preceded by adhesiolysis of the ampulla. Otherwise, direct traction on the tube will be needed to perform the surgical procedure. Dissection and section are then quite hazardous. Practically speaking, when it appears that the procedure will be simple, it should be carried out; otherwise, microsurgery should be planned, instead of an incomplete endosurgical procedure. Hereby, let us remind the reader that the infundibulum should never be grasped at the mucosal surface but always at its peritoneal surface. If traction is necessary, the grasp on the infundibulum should not be confined to only a part of it but rather to its entire circumference, so as to reduce the risk of injury.

Dense, broad adhesions between the ampulla and the ovary are a good indication for use of the CO_2 laser. The adhesion is brought under tension and progressively lysed by successive shots with a laser at a low wattage and with a slightly defocused beam. The beam is directed slightly toward the ovarian surface to avoid injury to the tube. In general, it is relatively easy to free the tube progressively from the ovary. In case of wide deperitonealized areas of the tube, the use of biologic glue is probably indicated to avoid recurrence of the adhesions.

Tubo-tubal adhesions

These adhesions can be easily missed unless a systematic exploration of the pelvis, with use of suprapubic instrumentation, is performed.

Filmy adhesions can form bridges from one segment of the tube to another. These bridges should be grasped with atraumatic forceps and resected with scissors. In most cases, this procedure is simple and without risk.

Conversely, dense adhesions are quite evident: the tube describes the sharp bends and convolutions. Those familiar with microsurgery know the difficulty of lysis of these adhesions; we therefore believe their resection should not be attempted endosurgically.

Ovarian adhesions (lateral aspects and broad ligament) (Figs. 9.21 and 9.22)

These adhesions suggest endometriosis, especially if they are isolated. Adhesiolysis of the ovary should be performed, because it is the only way to diagnose positively endometriotic lesions of the lateral aspect of the ovary.

Access to these adhesions is improved by grasping the ovarian ligament and applying an upward, rotating movement to the ovary. Adhesiolysis is then realized, either with previously described successive blunt dissection and section or by gently pushing the peritoneum of the broad ligament with half-closed scissors. For adhesions of type A and type B, this maneuver is very rewarding. However, for type C adhesions, one is very often faced with a deperitonealization of the posterior aspect of the broad ligament or with rupture of the ovarian cortex. We therefore consider that the treatment of this type of adhesion is somewhat illusory, but it must be done, at least partially, for diagnostic purposes.

In all cases, one must keep in mind that the ureter runs at the inferior aspect of these adhesions. Therefore one should be extremely careful to avoid injury. Hemostasis with electrocautery must be avoided as much as possible due to the proximity of the ureter.

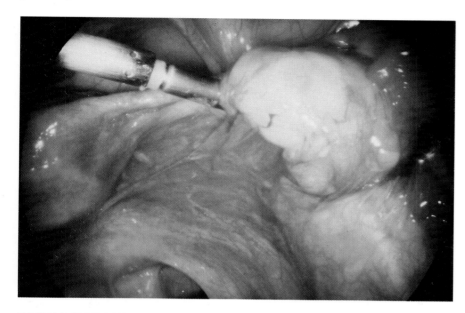

9.21 Retro-ovarian adhesions. This is a frequent site and can be diagnosed only through a two-puncture technique. Grasping the ovarian ligaments allows stretching and sectioning of the adhesions when they are filmy. This may not be successful in the case of dense adhesions.

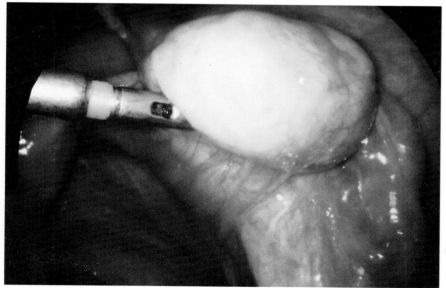

9.22 Alternative method for stretching retro-ovarian adhesions. Forceps are placed between the cranial pole of the ovary and the lateral pelvic wall, just underneath the infundibulopelvic ligament, and the ovary is gently pushed medially.

Adhesions of the cul-de-sac

These adhesions may involve various organs: uterus, tubes, ovaries, broad ligament, rectum—even ileum and omentum.

When the adhesions are filmy, treatment is easy. Elevation of the uterus is usually sufficient to put them under traction, followed by section close to the uterine surface.

Dense adhesions and obliteration of the cul-de-sac should not be operated on, especially if they extensively involve the bowel, because adhesiolysis in this case is dangerous and recurrence predictable. However, if no etiologic factor can be determined, adhesiolysis should be attempted in order to uncover possible endometriosis.

Utero-ovarian adhesions (Fig. 9.23)

These adhesions are almost always type C. Therefore adhesiolysis is very often difficult but never dangerous, and it may be the only possible way to diagnose endometriosis. The ovary is pushed laterally with forceps, whereas the uterine manipulator displaces the uterus contralaterally. Thereafter, adhesiolysis is performed, staying close to the ovary to reduce the risk of hemorrhage.

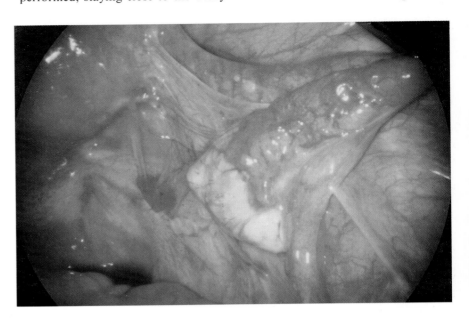

9.23 Adhesions between the uterine horn and ampulla are put under tension by traction on the tube. This maneuver also unveils filmy tubo-tubal adhesions.

Adhesions of omentum-abdominal wall (Fig. 9.24)

Sectioning of these adhesions is useful if it increases access to the pelvis. The omentum is pushed downward and adhesiolysis performed alongside the abdominal wall, because this is the cleavage plane, which allows bloodless dissection. Insertion of a second-puncture trocar, high on the abdominal wall, sometimes even at the level of the left hypochondrium, may aid approach of the adhesion with scissors at the appropriate angle. If an avascular cleavage plane cannot be identified, adhesiolysis should be performed step by step with prior bipolar coagulation.

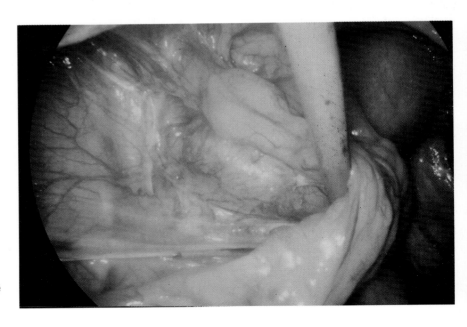

9.24 Adhesions between omentum and pelvic side wall are put under tension.

In addition, one should always check the anatomy behind the adhesion to avoid injury to the bowel: adhesions with the omentum usually consist of successive veils, which may mask a bowel loop attached to the abdominal wall. This visual inspection is more difficult at endoscopy, because exploration can be done only through a single angle of view.

Adhesions of bowel-genital tract

This adhesiolysis should be performed with the greatest care, whatever the type of adhesion involved.

Adhesions of omentum-genital tract

When only filmy adhesions are involved, the omentum can be lifted with an atraumatic forceps, and section of the adhesions is then relatively simple.

However, most often one deals with type C adhesions, which encase tubes and ovaries. Adhesiolysis is then performed by stabilizing the adnexae and by loosening the omentum with scissors in a half-open position, avoiding damage to the peritoneum of the pelvic organs. When a false cleavage plane is entered, when large areas of deperitonealization occur, or when bleeding is difficult to control, one should reevaluate whether the adhesiolysis should be continued.

Adhesions of bowel-genital tract

These adhesions can be sectioned if they are type A or type B. An atraumatic forceps is introduced between the bowel and the adnexa and the bowel is pushed away. Grasping the bowel should be avoided as much as possible. Sectioning of the adhesion is then performed, staying close along the ovary or tube.

Type C adhesions should not be dealt with and, in fact, constitute an absolute contraindication for endosurgical adhesiolysis. The risk of perforation outweighs the benefits.

Adhesions of cecum-abdominal wall

These adhesions are a sequela of appendectomy and are very often quite painful. Generally, they are easy to deal with and should be sectioned alongside the abdominal wall, either by simple section or by successive blunt dissection and section of the adhesions. Very often, one encounters successive veils of adhesions. These adhesions are generally avascular and should be differentiated from the mesenterium, which is richly vascularized. In case of dense adhesions, adhesiolysis is contraindicated, again because of the high risk of perforation. Frequently, atypical complaints of the patient will cease postoperatively.

Adhesions of bowel–bowel

Section of these adhesions is extremely difficult and should be considered only in the case of occlusion, due to mechanical ileus.

Adjuvant treatment

Adhesion formation and prevention of its recurrence remains an unsolved problem. Many adjuvant treatments have been proposed: corticoids, local or systemic; anti-inflammatory agents; colchicine; urokinase; and hypertonic solutions [16, 21, 22, 23, 27, 41, 43]. The only drug so far to show, objectively, any advantages in clinical trials is Dextran 70 [32]. 200 mL of this drug can be instilled at the end of the intervention. However, one should be aware of its complications.

In the future, we will probably see biocompatible glues play an important part in preventing the recurrence of adhesions. However, one should remember that no adjuvant treatment can replace an excellent technique or good evaluation of the type and etiology of the adhesions, both of which are of the utmost importance in the prevention of recurrence.

Complications of endosurgical adhesiolysis

Complications are uncommon for an experienced surgeon who knows his or her own limits and the contraindications for the procedure.

The more common complications are bowel injury and hemorrhage.

Bowel injuries

These are the most severe complications, but when diagnosed and treated promptly, they are without major consequences. However, when these lesions remain undiagnosed or occur secondary to, for example, electrocoagulation, they represent the principal cause of death following endosurgery.

It is therefore absolutely mandatory to visually inspect the entire abdominal cavity at the end of any endosurgical procedure, especially when the bowel has been involved and when electrical currrent has been used.

Hemorrhage

Infrequently, bleeding occurs at the level of the omentum, the mesosalpinx, or the infundibulopelvic ligament. These incidents are, of course, to be avoided, but hemostasis is possible in most cases through endosurgical techniques, either by application of electrocoagulation or with the use of ornithine-8-vasopressin.

It is most important to act quickly. Indeed, delay will lead to hematoma formation or even hemoperitoneum, which will make hemostasis even more difficult. Laparotomy rarely needs to be performed; however, if an injury of the infundibulopelvic ligament is not dealt with in the first 5 min, one should consider laparotomy, so as to avoid complications due to hypovolemia. This again emphasizes the necessity for a well-equipped operating room and service by personnel accustomed to both endoscopic and traditional surgical techniques.

Results of endosurgical adhesiolysis

Adhesiolysis and subsequent fertility

Let us consider four subgroups:
- Adhesiolysis only
- Adhesiolysis as part of a more complex operation
- Postoperative adhesiolysis
- Adhesiolysis in preparation for in vitro fertilization

Adhesiolysis only: one of the most rewarding endosurgical interventions [2, 5, 7, 9, 12, 19, 24, 36, 39, 45]

Table 9.3 summarizes the results reported in the literature. The success rate is very similar to that obtained by classical adhesiolysis via laparotomy. However, it is obvious that the postoperative course and cost-effectiveness favor laparoscopy.

In our experience, the majority of ectopic pregnancies occur within one year following adhesiolysis. When a pregnancy occurs after adhesiolysis, one should check its location, because approximately one in ten such pregnancies will be extrauterine. When a year has elapsed without conception, a second-look laparoscopy or in vitro fertilization (IVF) is warranted.

TABLE 9.3 **Results of adhesiolysis (sole procedure)**

Authors	Number of cases	IUP	%	EUP	%
Palmer, Madelenat [36]	144	42	29	11	7.6
Mintz [39]	65	24	37	7	11
Gomel [24]	92	57	62	5	5.4
Audebert [5]	50	15	30	0	
Abeille [2]	19	7	37	3	16
Mettler, Semm [38]	44	13	29		
Fayez [19]	50	30	60	2	4
Henry-Suchet [29]	38	15	39	1	3
Bruhat et al. [9]	93	48	51	7	5

Preoperative adhesiolysis

The impact of preoperative adhesiolysis on the outcome of microsurgery has not been studied thus far, but most microsurgeons perform preoperative endosurgical adhesiolysis [5, 19, 25]. Adhesiolysis has several advantages:

− It permits complete exploration of the pelvis and, hence, a thorough evaluation of the extent of the lesions.

− It facilitates evaluation of the prognosis, which, in turn, influences the selection of patients for either microsurgery or in vitro fertilization (see Chapter 10).

− It permits evaluation of the histology of the adhesions and the cytology of the peritoneal fluid, so one can institute antibiotic and/or anti-inflammatory treatment prior to the intervention.

− Finally, it facilitates the subsequent intervention by shortening the time required for microsurgical adhesiolysis or even totally eliminating the need for it.

Our own data (unpublished) on 78 adnexa show that regression occurred in 48 cases (61.5 %) and recurrence has been observed in 30 cases (38.5 %). This rather high recurrence rate can be explained by the fact that many patients have progressive lesions. However, the outcome of tubal microsurgery depends on the extent of adhesions at the time of surgery [37]. Therefore, it is likely that preoperative endosurgical adhesiolysis will have a positive impact on the outcome of the microsurgical procedure. To our knowledge, there are no data available in the literature on the subject.

Postoperative adhesiolysis

Most microsurgeons perform this type of operation. Microsurgical interventions are subject to adhesion recurrence or to primary formation of adhesions. Various studies have demonstrated that the best timing for postoperative adhesiolysis is between 6 and 10 weeks after the primary intervention [18, 42]. Our own data suggest that 20% of pregnancies after microsurgery would not have occurred without postoperative adhesiolysis. However, randomized comparative studies are not available; thus, conclusions remain subjective.

In vitro fertilization

Adhesiolysis facilitates access to the ovary prior to puncture of the follicle. More recently, ultrasonographic guidance has received a great deal of attention. Nonetheless, adhesiolysis remains important in view of the need for exact diagnosis and subsequent choice of appropriate treatment. Finally, an ovary free of adhesions functions considerably better than an ovary encapsulated in dense adhesions.

Adhesiolysis for pelvic pain

The relationship between adhesions and pelvic pain remains uncertain, probably because it is inconsistent. Adhesiolysis certainly improves the symptomatology of a number of patients; however, it is difficult to exclude the placebo effect [44]. The physiopathology of pain due to adhesions is not always clear. Clinical examination remains the most important element in considering operative lysis of adhesions for treatment of pelvic pain.

All adhesions do not cause pain (e.g., the adhesions between the tube and peritoneum, tube and ovary, and tube and omentum). However, when adhesions encapsulate the ovary, they can be the source of pain due to ovarian dysfunction [1]. Also, many adhesions following appendectomy involve the bowel and may seem to cause pain due to phenomena of traction, torsion, or subocclusion. Finally, fixed retroversion may be extremely painful. All these situations justify adhesiolysis, which may uncover endometriosis and which is mandatory prior to, for example, performance of an antefixation (see Chapter 15).

Conclusion

Adhesiolysis is one of the most frequently performed endosurgical procedures. Its possibilities are tremendous provided that the operator uses adequate equipment and follows a well-defined, standardized technique with several suprapubic puncture sites. The usefulness of laparoscopy in pure adhesiolysis requires no further debate. However, as a complement to tubal microsurgery, its value still needs to be established, although many factors argue in its favor. It should also be noted, however, that many procedures formerly requiring microsurgery, such as fimbrioplasty and salpingostomy, are now increasingly being handled via endosurgery.

References

1. Abeille J.P., « La dystrophie ovarienne *par en dehors* », *Contrac. Fertil. Sexual*, 1983; Suppl. 11 (3) : 557-562.
2. Abeille J.P., « La place de l'adhésiolyse per-cœlioscopique dans les infections pelviennes aiguës », Journée du Collège National des Cœlioscopistes Français, Paris, 5-6 décembre 1981.
3. Adhesion study group, « Reduction of postoperative pelvic adhesions with intraperitoneal, 32 % Dextran 70 », *Fertil. Steril.*, 1983; 40 : 612.
4. Allis H., « The cause and prevention of postoperative intraperitoneal adhesions », *Surg. Gynecol. Obstet.*, 1971; 133 : 497.
5. Audebert A., Emperaire J.C., « Chirurgie tubaire et fonction ovarienne », *Contrac. Fertil. Sexual.*, 1983; 11 (1) : 35.
6. Audebert A., « L'adhésiolyse per-cœlioscopique », *Contrac. Fertil. Sexual.*, 1983; 11 (6) : 857-862.
7. Bercovici B., Gailly R., « The cytology of the human peritoneal fluid », *Acta Cytol.*, 1978; 32 : 124.

8. Bronson R.A., Wallach E.E., « Lysis of periadnexal adhesions for correction of infertility », *Fertil. Steril.*, 1977; 28 (6) : 613.

9. Bruhat M.A., Mage G., Manhes H., Pouly J.L., Jacquetin B., « Place de la cœlioscopie dans le bilan de la stérilité féminine », *J. Gynecol. Biol. Reprod.*, 1980; 9 : 337.

10. Bruhat M.A., Mage G., Manhes H., Soualhat C., Ropert J.F., Pouly J.L., « Laparoscopic procedures to promote fertility. Ovariolysis and salpingolysis. Results of 93 selected cases », *Acta Eur. Fertil.*, 1983; 14 : 2.

11. Buttram V.C., Vaquero C., « Post-ovarian wedge resection adhesive disease », *Fertil. Steril.*, 1975; 26 : 874.

12. Capsi E., Halperin Y., Bukovsky J., « The importance of periadnexal adhesions in tubal reconstructive surgery for infertility », *Fertil. Steril.*, 1979; 31 : 296.

13. Daniell J.F., Pittaway D.E., Maxson W.S., « The role of laparoscopic adhesiolysis in an *in vitro* fertilization program », *Fertil. Steril.*, 1983; 40 (1) : 49.

14. Dargent D., « Les stérilités tubaires iatrogènes ou pitié pour les trompes »; In: Oviducte et fertilité, Masson, Paris, 1979; 421.

15. De Brux J., Dupre-Froment J., Mintz M., « Cytology of the peritoneal fluid sampled by coelioscopic or by cul-de-sac puncture », *Acta Cytol.*, 1968; 12 : 395.

16. De Brux J., Mintz M., « Explorations cyto- et histopathologiques du péritoine pelvien. Le tissu cellulaire pelvien », Masson, Paris, 1973; 133.

17. Dizerega G.S., Hodgen G.D., « Prevention of postoperative tubal adhesions. Comparative study of commonly used agents », *Fertil. Gynecol.*, 1980; 136 (2) : 173.

18. Donnez J., Thomas K., « Luteal fonction after tubal sterilization », *Obstet. Gynecol.*, 1981; 57 : 65.

19. Dubuisson J.B., Barbot J., Henrion R., « La cœlioscopie de contrôle précoce après microchirurgie tubaire », *J. Gynecol. Obstet. Biol. Reprod.*, 1979; 8 : 655.

20. Fayez J.A., « An assessment of the role of operative laparoscopy in tuboplasty », *Fertil. Steril.*, 1983; 39 (4) : 476.

21. Fredericks C.M., Anderson W.R., « The effect of transaction of the accessory ligaments on reproduction in the rabbit », *Fertil. Steril.*, 1979; 32 (2) : 219.

22. Gervin A.S., Pucket C.L., Silver D., « Serosal hypofribrinolysis. A cause of postoperative adhesions », *Am. J. Surg.*, 1973; 125 : 80.

23. Gilmore O.J.A., Reid C., « Noxythiolin and peritoneal adhesion formation », *Br. J. Surg.*, 1976; 63 : 978.

24. Glucksman D.L., Warren W.D., « The effect of topically applied corticosteroids in the prevention of peritoneal adhesions », *Surgery*, 1966; 60 : 352.

25. Gomel V., « Salpingo-ovariolysis by laparoscopy in infertility », *Fertil. Steril.*, 1983; 40 (5) : 607.

26. Gomel V., « Classification of operations for tubal and peritoneal factors causing infertility », *Clin. Obstet. Gynaecol.*, 1980; 23 (4) : 1259.

27. Gordji M., Palmer R., « Etude statistique des causes des adhérences pelviennes dans 250 cas vérifiés par la cœlioscopie », *Bull. Soc. Fr. Gynecol.*, 1968; 38 : 51.

28. Grobety V.J., « Les adhérences postopératoires », Thèse, Genève, 1972.

29. Henry-Suchet J., Loffredo V., « Traitement chirurgical des stérilités tubaires: Intérêt de la greffe de péritoine libre et de la cœlioscopie précoce dans la prévention des adhérences », *Nouv. Presse Med.*, 1980; 9 (5) : 311.

30. Henry-Suchet J., Gadras P., Loffredo V., « Ovario-salpingolyse cœlioscopique. A propos d'une série de 120 cas dont 63 pour stérilité », *Gynécologie*, 1979; 30 (2) : 119.

31. Hulka J.F., « Classification of adnexal adhesions: a proposal and evaluation of its prognostic value », *Fertil. Steril*, 1978; 30 : 661.

32. Hulka J.F., « Adnexal adhesions: a prognostic staging and classification system based on a five-year survey of fertility surgery results at Chapel Hill, North Carolina », *Am. J. Obstet. Gynecol.*, 1982; 144 (2) : 141.

33. Jacobson L., Weström L., « Objectivized diagnosis of acute pelvic inflammatory disease », *Am. J. Obstet. Gynecol.*, 1969; 105 : 1088.

34. Jessen H., « Forty-five operations for sterilty », *Acta Obstet. Gynecol. Scand.*, 1971; 50 : 105.

35. Mac Gowan L., Bunnag B., « A morphological classification of peritoneal fluid cytology in women », *Int. J. Gynaecol. Obstet.*, 1973; 11 : 173.

36. Madelenat P., Palmer R., « Etude critique des libérations per-cœlioscopiques des adhérences péri-annexielles », *J. Gynecol. Obstet. Biol. Reprod.*, 1973; 8 : 347.

37. Mage G., Pouly J.L., Bouquet de La Jolinière J., Chabrand S., Bruhat M.A., « Obstructions tubaires distales: microchirurgie ou fécondation *in vitro* », *J. Gynecol. Obstet. Biol. Reprod.*, 1984; 13 : 933-937.

38. Mettler L., Giesez H., Semm K., « Treatment of female infertility due to tubal obstruction by operative laparoscopy », *Fertil. Steril.*, 1979; 32 : 43.

39. Mintz M., « La libération par cœlioscopie d'adhérences dans 55 cas de stérilité féminine. Technique, résultats, indications », *Gynécologie*, 1985; 26 (4) : 277.

40. Palmer R., « La cœlioscopie dans le diagnostic et le traitement des adhérences pelviennes », *Contract. Fertil. Sexual.*, 1980; 7 (11) : 797.

41. Querleu D., « Le traitement péri-opératoire des adhésiolyses pelviennes », *Gynécologie*, 1983; 34 : 35.

42. Raj S., Hulka J., « Second look laparoscopy in infertility surgery therapeutic and prognostic value », *Fertil. Steril.*, 1982; 38 (3) : 325.

43. Replogle R., Johnson R., Gross R. E., « Prevention of postoperative intestinal adhesions with combined promethazine and dexamethazone therapy: experimental and clinical studies », *Ann. Surg.*, 1966; 163 : 580.

44. Rudigoz R. C., « Fréquence dans la population générale des lésions infracliniques supposées algogènes », XXes Assises de la Société Française de Gynécologie, Clermont-Ferrand, 28–29–30 mai 1981, Masson, Paris.

45. Semm K., Mettler L., « Technical progress in pelvic surgery via operative laparoscopy », *Am. J. Obstet. Gynecol.*, 1980; 138 (2) : 121.

46. Young P. E., Egan J. E., Barlow J. J., Mulligan W. J., « Reconstructive surgery for infertility at the Boston Hospital for women », *Am. J. Obstet. Gynecol.*, 1970; 108 : 1092.

10

Salpingostomy

Endosurgical salpingostomy was first performed a long time ago [4]. After being somewhat abandoned, better equipment and the CO_2 laser have brought about a revival of the procedure. Patient selection and long-standing experience are the mainstays of success for this rather difficult procedure.

Introduction

During the seventies, reconstructive surgery of the fallopian tube was proscribed by the proponents of microsurgery [12]. However, refinements in surgical technique did not improve the results of salpingostomy, in contrast to those of reanastomosis [11, 12]. These data reconfirm that the most important factor for success of reconstructive surgery is the status of the tube itself [3, 6]. In the meantime, the eighties have seen the development of three phenomena: technical improvement of laparoscopy, development of the CO_2 laser [1, 5], and in vitro fertilization.

Today, the choice is between IVF and reconstructive surgery [5]. Hysterosalpingography and laparoscopy establish the selection. In cases with good prognosis, endoscopy can be extended to encompass treatments such as salpingostomy and fimbrioplasty. In unfavorable cases, IVF is advisable.

Procedure

Instrumentation

Ideally, the CO_2 laser is used for incision and eversion of the fimbriated end of the tube. In addition, some atraumatic graspers and forceps are required. Even without the CO_2 laser, it is feasible to perform a salpingostomy.

Transcervical chromopertubation is used to distend the tube with relatively high pressure. Two suprapubic trocars are used. When the CO_2 laser is involved, a third suprapubic incision is required in the midline, some 3 to 4 cm higher than the other incisions. The laser can also be introduced through the operating channel of the laparoscope.

Adhesiolysis

Adhesiolysis is always performed first. This is quite important, because it establishes the conditions for good access to the fimbriated end of the fallopian tube. Two situations are commonly encountered.

– Veil-like adhesions that can easily be transected, so that the tube, as well as the ovary, is readily mobilized. This allows recovery of tubal mobility with regard to the ovarian surface, a very important parameter for success.

– Dense adhesions that require more precautions, as explained in Chapter 9. If it is feasible to free the fallopian tube, especially from the ovarian surface, then the procedure is undertaken. If not, the intervention is aborted in favor of subsequent microsurgery or IVF, according to the general condition of the pelvic organs. In our experience, when endosurgical intervention was impractical, it proved to be a difficult microsurgical case, and we therefore tend to opt for IVF in these cases.

Tuboplasty

Endosurgical techniques do not differ in essence from those applied during microsurgery. Experience in microsurgery is helpful in performing laparoscopic procedures. Tubal anatomy determines whether one opts for fimbrioplasty or salpingostomy.

Fimbrioplasty

Because the distal opening of the tube is still recognizable, the anatomy is easily restored. Theoretically, the surgery involves only the serosa and is relatively simple to perform. This technique is applied in cases of phimosis and where the mucosal folds can still be recognized. The technique consists of resection of the constricted serosa and dilation of the ostium. The laser does not offer any advantage over the common endosurgical equipment unless eversion is required—which should, in principle, not be the case. The tube is grasped through the ipsilateral trocar with an atraumatic forceps at the ampullary serosa. A second forceps, inserted through the contralateral trocar, is used to grasp the veil-like adhesions, which are gradually peeled off the fimbriated end and resected. Sometimes it is easier to introduce an atraumatic forceps into the ostium and to gently spread its long jaws, rupturing the adhesions. Occasionally, scissors or the CO_2 laser are required to complete this maneuver.

Once the fimbrioplasty is performed, chromopertubation shows free passage without terminal dilation of the ampulla. In all cases, one should search for adhesions connecting mucosal folds, and these should be resected. The search can be done with an atraumatic forceps or a flexible tuboscope. This type of fimbrioplasty is usually relatively easy and in most cases requires no hemostasis.

Salpingostomy

Salpingostomy is the creation of a new tubal orifice as close to its anatomic location as possible. The tube is generally completely occluded, or occasionally has a fistulous tract. Salpingostomy requires incision through all the layers of the oviduct, not just the serosa, as was the case in fimbrioplasty. Eversion of the

edges is almost always necessary. The CO_2 laser is quite handy for these interventions, which encompass three steps:
- Opening the hydrosalpinx
- Incision of the wall
- Eversion

Opening the hydrosalpinx (Figs. 10.1 through 10.6)

This can be done in several ways. First, transcervical injection of methylene blue distends the tube. An atraumatic forceps stabilizes the tube at approximately 2 cm from its end. The previous orifice can be located by visualizing the starlike scar at the tubal end. The CO_2 laser ($20,000 \ W/cm^2$) opens the tube at the level of the previous ostium. Otherwise, one can also increase the intratubal pressure, which quite often leads to rupture of the tube at the previous orifice, which is the site of least resistance.

Incision of the wall

Ideally, three to four radial incisions are made from the opening to the periphery over 1 to 2 cm, depending on the diameter of the hydrosalpinx. The first incision should be directed toward the ovary.

With CO_2 laser: Two atraumatic forceps grasp the tube at its end, close to the opening previously made. The first incision with focused beam ($20,000 \ W/cm^2$) is directed toward the ovary. Then, two or three more incisions are made radially from the initial opening on the course of the scar if visualized. Hemostasis is unnecessary (Figs. 10.7 through 10.12).

Without CO_2 laser: The technique can be identical, using scissors and bipolar coagulation if required. One can also proceed by gentle traction with two atraumatic forceps. First the initial opening is widened by introducing an atraumatic forceps into the tubal lumen and spreading its jaws. Then the edges are grasped at opposing points and traction is used to open the fimbriated end still further. This is repeated three to four times in order to create a corresponding number of fringes. Hemostasis, if required, is done with bipolar forceps. This technique is rather difficult to describe but easily understood by those who have performed salpingostomies using microsurgical techniques (Figs. 10.13 through 10.15).

Eversion

Suturing is not mandatory. Eversion is obtained by coagulation of the serosal surface with defocused laser beam [8] at low intensity ($500 \ W/cm^2$) (Figs. 10.16 through 10.19). Eversion is due to retraction of the serosa caused by the superficial coagulation. This eversion is permanent and easy to perform when the tubal wall is thin and supple. The CO_2 laser can be replaced by bipolar coagulation at low intensity (Figs. 10.20 through 10.24).

As for fimbrioplasty, it is advisable to look for adhesions between mucosal folds. Duration of the intervention depends on the site and on the experience of the operator—on average, 30 to 60 min. The CO_2 laser eases accomplishing the eversion.

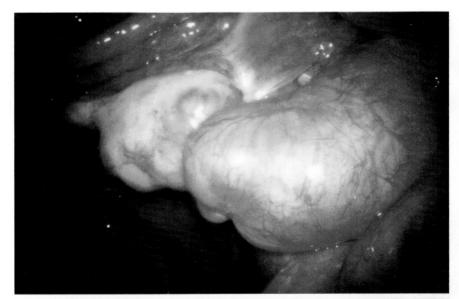

10.1 Hydrosalpinx, stage 2.

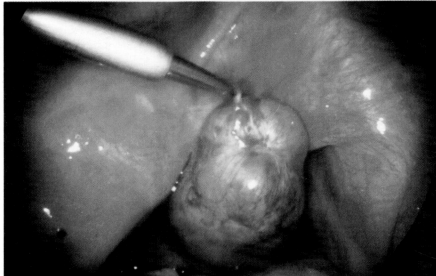

10.2 Chromopertubation causes the hydrosalpinx to distend. This facilitates localization of the scar at the distal end. Increase of the intratubal pressure sometimes leads to spontaneous rupture of the hydrosalpinx at the level of its (occluded) ostium.

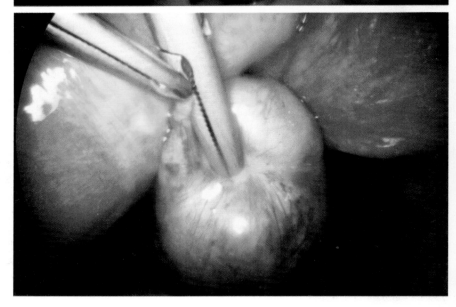

10.3 An atraumatic grasper is introduced into the small opening.

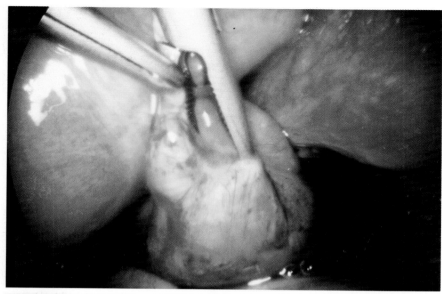

10.4 Blunt opening of the graspers forces the hydrosalpinx to open. The fibrous tissue which bridges between the mucosal folds will rupture without damage to the tubal wall. This procedure is completely bloodless.

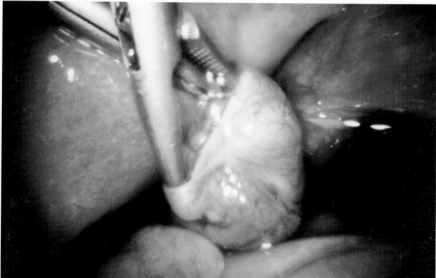

10.5 This figure illustrates well how the fibrous bridges are put under tension and ruptured.

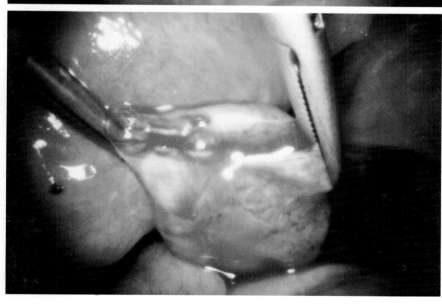

10.6 Rupture of the fibrous bridges is completed by applying two graspers, pulling in opposite directions.

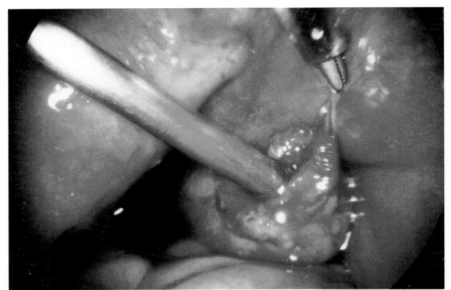

10.7 The tubal lumen is then rinsed.

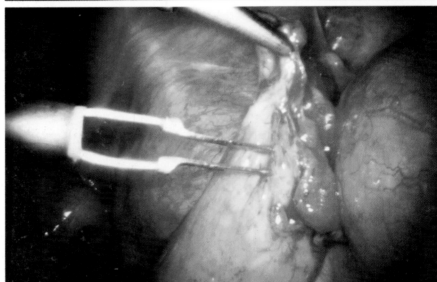

10.8–10.11 Eversion of the fimbriated end is obtained with bipolar coagulation. A low-intensity current is used to avoid extensive damage to the tubal wall. Shrinkage of the serosal surface causes eversion of the fimbriated end.

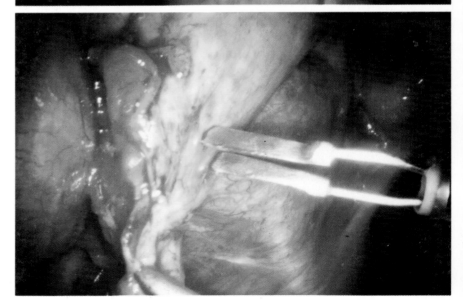

10.9

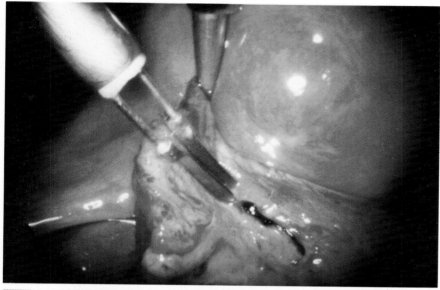

10.10

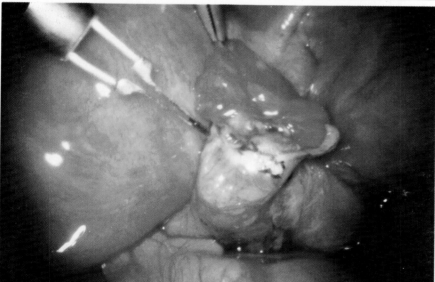

10.11

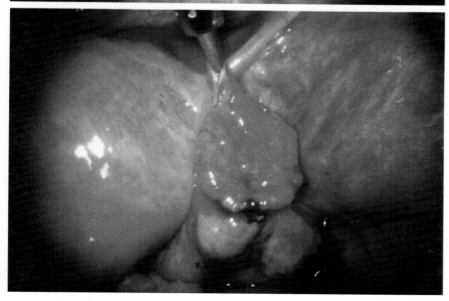

10.12 Final aspect of the fimbriated end.

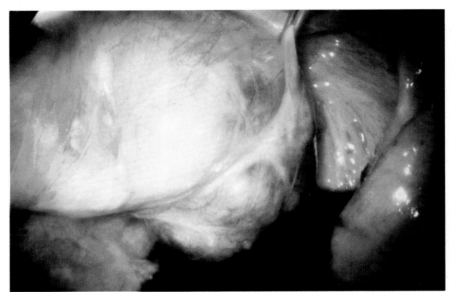

10.13 Hydrosalpinx.

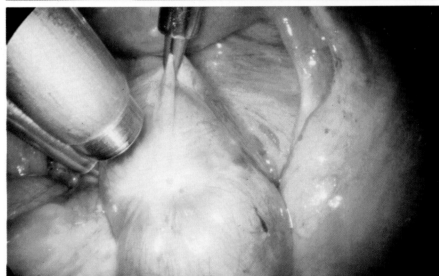

10.14 Hydrotubation is performed to locate the scar. Using the CO_2 laser, it is advisable to avoid high pressures during hydrotubation, because premature collapse of the tube would hamper the use of the laser. It is preferable to make several shallow incisions prior to opening the hydrosalpinx.

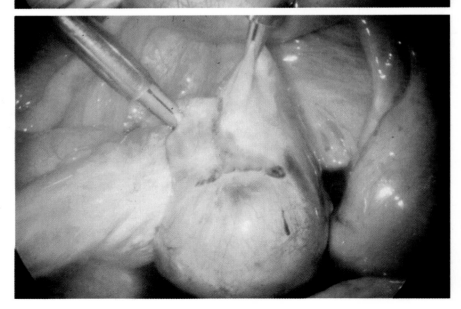

10.15–10.18 A stellar incision is performed, similar to the procedure done at laparotomy. The CO_2 laser seals small vessels, making the surgery almost completely bloodless. The oviduct is stablized with two atraumatic graspers.

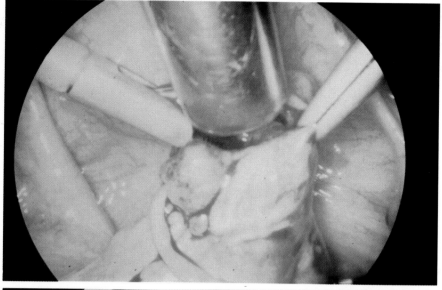

10.16

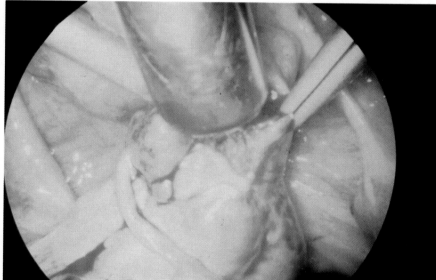

10.17

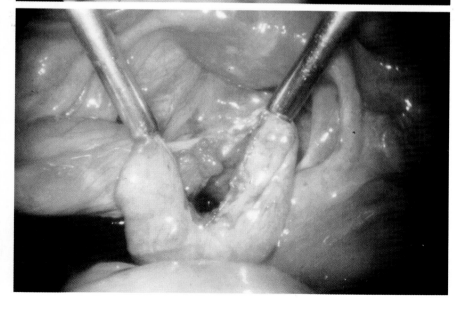

10.18

10.19–10.20 The incision of the fimbriated end is completed by applying traction with two atraumatic graspers. In the end, the fimbria-ovarica is reconstructed.

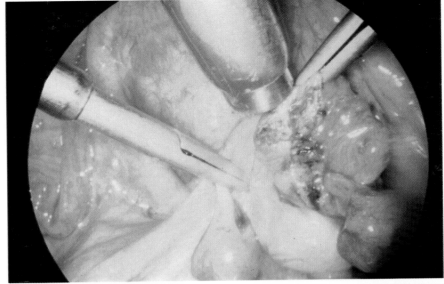

10.19

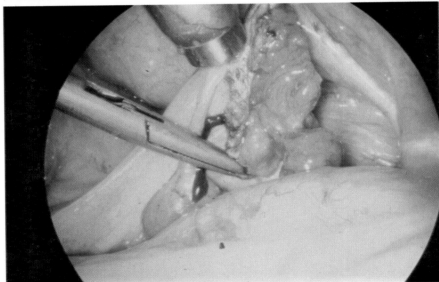

10.20

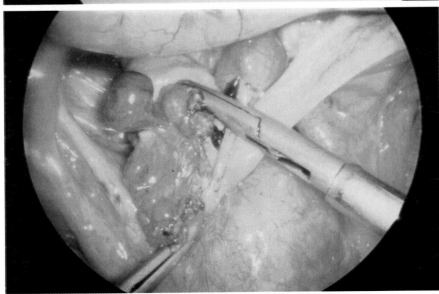

10.21–10.23 Using the defocused CO_2 laser, one can cause retraction ("hatching") of the serosal edges.

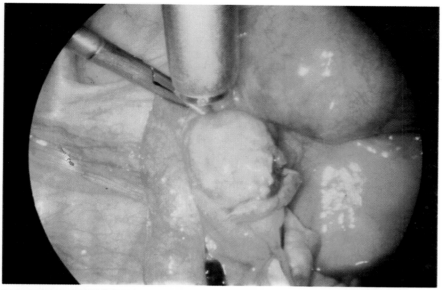

10.22

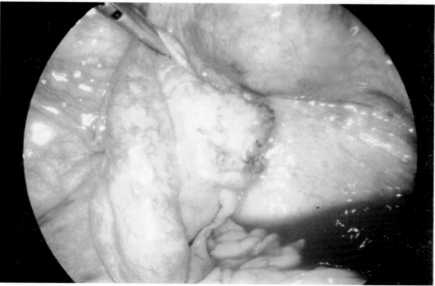

10.23

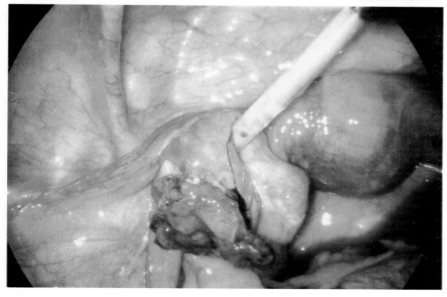

10.24 Aspect of the fimbriated end at completion of the procedure. A hydrotubation with Methylene blue is performed.

Results

Table 10.1 represents the results of the first 87 patients on whom we performed surgery. An intrauterine pregnancy (IUP) occurred in 29 patients (33.3 %) and extrauterine pregnancy (EUP) in 6 (6.9 %). These results are comparable to the results obtained by microsurgery in 76 patients (Table 10.2). Obviously the advantages of the laparoscopic approach are reduced hospital stay, less trauma to the abdominal wall, and the combination of diagnosis and treatment within one intervention. These advantages are most obvious when dealing with patients who have had multiple invasive diagnostic tests and surgical interventions.

TABLE 10.1 **Fertility outcome after laparoscopic salpingostomy (author's data)**

Stages	N	%	Intrauterine Pregnancy		Extrauterine Pregnancy	
			N	%	N	%
Stage I	22	32.36	10	44.5	1	4.5
Stage II	27	39.70	6	22.2	4	14.8
Stage III	13	19.12	1	7.7	0	0
Stage IV	6	8.9	0	0	0	0
Total	68		17	25	5	7.4

TABLE 10.2 **Fertility outcome after microsurgical salpingostomy (author's data)**

Stages	Number of cases	IUP		EUP	
		Number	%	Number	%
Tube					
Stage I	12	7	58.3	1	8.3
Stage II	30	11	36.6	3	10.0
Stage III	21	2	9.5	3	14.2
Stage IV	13	0	0	0	0
Total	76	20	26.3	7	9.2
Adhesions					
Stage 0	18	7	38.8	3	16.6
Stage I	25	8	32.0	0	0
Stage II	15	4	26.6	1	6.6
Stage III	18	1	5.5	3	16.6
Total	76	20	26.3	7	9.2

Indications

Laparoscopy for salpingostomy is performed in cases of distal tubal occlusion, usually due to infection, when one is sure that there is no longer any inflammation present. It is of utmost importance to search for the presence of possible chronic *Chlamydia* infection. Serologic determination of antibody titer will select patients at risk for carrying a chronic infection. In these cases, a 4-week course of antibiotics should precede the surgery.

Should one always operate on distal tubal occlusion? The answer to this question is essentially dependent on the status of the fallopian tube. The most sophisticated technique cannot overcome this limitation, but of course a bad technique could ruin whatever little chance there is. As for microsurgery, careful patient selection is essential. Fimbrioplasty bears an excellent prognosis in that patient selection is less critical. The surgery itself is relatively easy, and we consider it part of the adhesiolysis. The prognosis is excellent—on the order of 30 to 35 % according to data in the literature [2, 10]. Laparotomy for the purpose of fimbrioplasty has always appeared disproportional to us, and we therefore rarely performed it.

Salpingostomy has a less favorable prognosis: 33.3 % in our endoscopy series and 26.3 % in our microsurgery cases. Therefore careful patient selection is required. We have designed a scoring system, based on the results of hysterosalpingography and diagnostic laparoscopy, allowing us to select patients either for surgical treatment or IVF [9]. This scoring system integrates data relating to tubal patency, aspects of the tubal mucosa, and the tubal wall (Table 10.3). The lesions can then be classified into four stages, from more favorable to less favorable. In our microsurgical salpingostomy series, the success rate of the surgery was 58.3 %, 36.6 %, 9.5 %, and 0 % in stages I, II, III, and IV, respectively (Table 10.2). When the tubal and adhesion scoring systems are combined (Table 10.4), one can distinguish two main groups of patients. The first group includes stages I and II with no, few, or a moderate number of adhesions. The success rate in these patients is 50 %, with an 8.8 % rate of ectopic pregnancy. These are the candidates for endosurgical salpingostomy. The second group are those patients with a tubal score in categories III and IV

TABLE 10.3 **Staging of distal tubal disease**

Patency	Mucosal folds	Tubal wall
	Well preserved **0**	Normal **0**
Phimosis **2**	Decreased **5**	Thin **5**
Hydrosalpinx **5**	Absent or follicular salpingitis **10**	Thickened or fibrosed **10**

Note: Stage I = 2–5; stage II = 6–10; stage III = 11–15; stage IV > 15.

TABLE 10.4 **Choice: surgery versus IVF (microsurgery data)**

	Number of cases	IUP	EUP
Tubal score I, II; adhesion score 0, I, II	34	17 (50 %)	3 (8.8 %)
Tubal score III, IV; adhesion score III	42	3 (7 %)	4 (9.5 %)

and those with severe adhesions, independent of the tubal score. The success rate here is only 7 % with a 9.5 % rate of ectopic pregnancy. In these cases, we advise IVF.

Our data on patients operated on via laparoscopy give similar figures: 50 % in stage I, 32.4 % in stage II, and 8.3 % in stage III. In conclusion, the selection of patients for laparoscopic salpingostomy is similar to that for microsurgery.

It is too early to state that laparoscopic interventions lead to similar results, using the same measures as for microsurgery, although our data seem to indicate so. The data in the literature are inconclusive. Mettler [10] reports 26 % success in 38 cases, Fayez [2] 0 % in 19 cases, Gomel [4] 44 % in 9 cases, and Lauritzen [7] 13 % in 23 cases. These authors did not use the CO_2 laser. Daniell and Herbert [1] report a 22.7 % success rate in their first series with CO_2 laser. These series concern too small a number of patients for definitive conclusions. In addition, some series [7] involved patients who had previously had a tuboplasty performed.

Conclusion

Laparoscopic salpingostomy is not always easy. It requires experience in both laparoscopy and tubal surgery. One should also consider that a mistake in technique can lead to disastrous consequences, and this in a patient who was considered to have a good chance for success. Recourse to IVF "in the back of the mind" should not be an excuse for less than excellent surgical technique.

References

1. Daniell J.F., Herbert C.M., « Laparoscopic salpingostomy utilizing the carbon dioxide laser », *Fertil. Steril.*, 1984; 41 : 558.
2. Fayez J.A., « An assessment of the role of operative laparoscopy in tuboplasty », *Fertil. Steril.*, 1983; 39 : 476.
3. Frantzen C., Schlosser H.W., « Microsurgery and post-infectious tubal infertility », *Fertil. Steril.*, 1982; 38 : 397.
4. Gomel V., « Salpingostomy by laparoscopy », *J. Reprod. Med.*, 1977; 18 : 265.
5. Hedon B., Denjean R., Damies J.P., Mares P., Valentin B., Viala J.L., Durang G., « Stérilités tubaires : fécondation in vitro ou microchirurgie », *Presse Med.*, 1984; 13 : 33.
6. Hulka J.F., « Adnexal adhesions : a prognostic staging and classification system based on a five year survey of fertility surgery results at Chapel Hill, North Carolina », *Am. J. Obstet. Gynecol.*, 1982; 144 : 141.
7. Lauritzen J.G., Pagel J.D., Vangsted P., Starup J., « Result of repeated tuboplasties », *Fertil. Steril.*, 1983; 40 : 472.
8. Mage G., Bruhat M.A., « Pregnancy following salpingostomy : comparison between carbon dioxide laser and electrosurgery procedures », *Fertil. Steril.*, 1983; 40 : 472.
9. Mage G., Pouly J.L., Bouquet de Jolinière J., Chabrand S., Riouallon A., Bruhat, M.A., « A preoperative classification to predict the intrauterine and ectopic pregnancy rates after distal tubal microsurgery », *Fertil. Steril.*, 1986; 46 : 807.
10. Mettler L., Giesel H., Semm K., « Treatment of female infertility due to tubal obstruction by operative laparoscopy », *Fertil. Steril.*, 1979; 32 : 384.
11. Musich J.R., Behrman S.J., « Surgical management of tubal obstruction of the uterotubal junction », *Fertil. Steril.*, 1983; 40 : 423.
12. Winston R.M.L., « Microsurgery of the Fallopian tube : from fantasy to reality », *Fertil. Steril.*, 1980; 34 : 521.

11
Endometriosis

Endoscopy has two distinct purposes:
- Diagnosis. This aspect encompasses initial diagnosis, staging, second look, evaluation of recurrence or sequelae.
- Treatment. This aspect of endoscopy has become increasingly important since the introduction of the CO_2 laser.

Introduction

Clinical diagnosis of pelvic endometriosis is difficult because
- Symptoms can be attributed to many gynecologic diseases.
- There is a low correlation between physical examination and extent of disease [38].
- There is a large incidence of asymptomatic disease (10 to 40 % [1, 5, 16, 30]).
- Follow-up to determine progression of disease is difficult.

Diagnosis requires surgical exploration and histology. Laparoscopy drastically changed our attitude toward evaluation of the disease. However, one should be prepared to puncture an even slightly enlarged ovary or to perform adhesiolysis for release of ovary or tube from the pelvic wall in order to uncover lesions on the inner surface of the ovary, which are easily masked by the adhesions they generate.

Laparoscopic diagnosis

Common endometriotic lesions

Peritoneal implants (Figs. 11.1 through 11.5)

The typical lesion is the so-called powder-burned small cyst—brown, blue, or almost black and 2 to 5 mm in diameter. They are surrounded by a peritoneal reaction such as the pathognomonic starlike scar. Other lesions are red, slightly brown, flat as opposed to cystic, and variable in extent as well as irregular in contour. It seems that the darker these lesions are and the more they are surrounded by large areas of sclerosis, the less likely it is that hormonally active endometrial tissue will be found on biopsy [13].

One should note that
- Red implants and some clear vesicles (1 to 2 mm) on the peritoneal surface usually represent endometriosis.
- Biopsies of apparently healthy peritoneum surrounding typical lesions and at the level of peritoneal defects (erroneously called the *Allen and Masters syndrome*) sometimes show the presence of endometriosis.

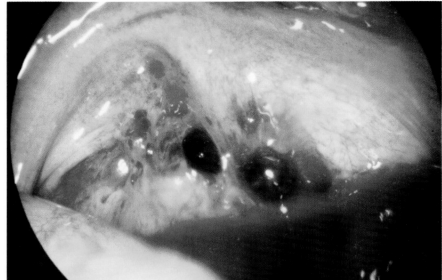

11.1 Typical appearance of peritoneal implants, the variation of which is greater than what is classically taught.

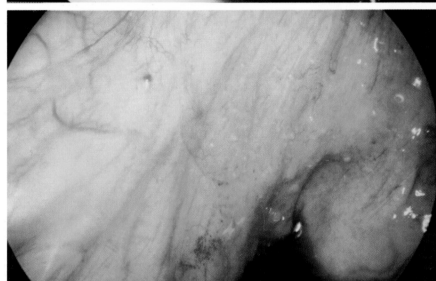

11.2 Small translucent vesicular lesions of the peritoneum should encourage the surgeon to perform a close survey of the peritoneal surface. A biopsy is strongly advised, even though a hemorrhagic lesion nearby brings to mind the possibility of endometriosis.

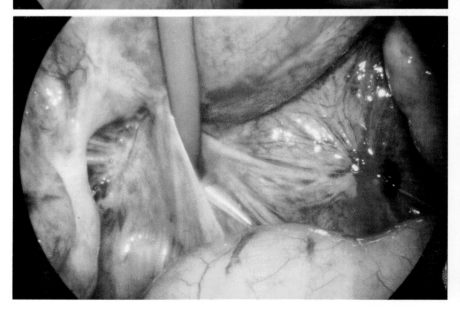

11.3 Peritoneal fibrosis appears quite typically as a stellar retraction (right side of the illustration). The left side shows an example of how endometriosis causes partial occlusion of the cul-de-sac with the peritoneal scarring appearing as a sickle.

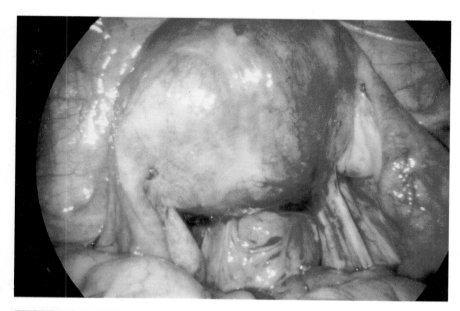

11.4 Another example of a sicklelike peritoneal fibrosis, leading to obliteration of the cul-de-sac. This aspect may correspond merely to scarring, but a search for active lesions is indicated.

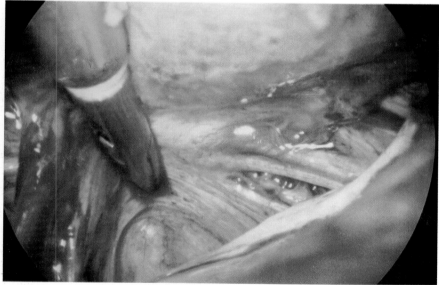

11.5 An example of a peritoneal defect, falsely labeled the Allen and Masters syndrome. In actuality this appearance of the peritoneum is linked to the presence of endometriosis, as was demonstrated by Chatman. The vascular anomalies seen lateral from the lesion are remindful of the disease. Here, too, a biopsy is recommended.

Adhesions (Figs. 11.6 and 11.7)

The most characteristic presentation is obliteration of the cul-de-sac and broad adhesions between the ovary and the posterior aspect of the uterus and between the ovary and broad ligament.

Endometriosis can also cause filmy adhesions. If they contain multiple vessels with petechiae, histology may sometimes show the presence of active endometriosis.

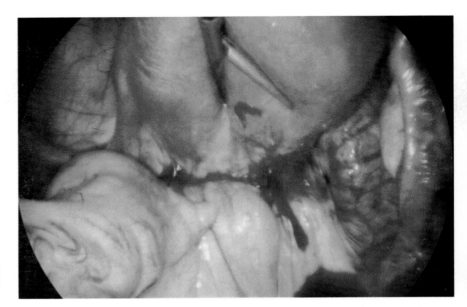

11.6 Total obliteration of the cul-de-sac due to adherence of the rectum to the posterior aspect of the uterus, a quite typical view.

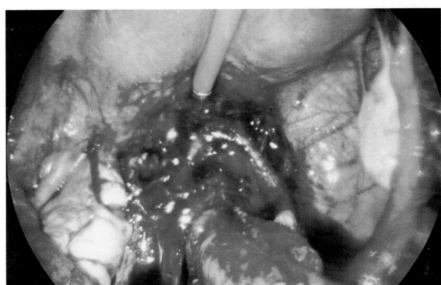

11.7 Adhesiolysis uncovers the endometriotic lesions. This maneuver is only feasible in case of active lesions. When fibrosis is prominent, adhesiolysis may reveal to be dangerous.

Ovarian lesions (Figs. 11.8 through 11.14)

Small lesions, similar to those on the peritoneum, are easily identified provided all surfaces of the ovary are accessible. Less obvious is the diagnosis of small cysts (2 to 3 cm) which are encapsulated in the ovary, causing only minimal enlargement and distinguishable only by a brown-stained scar on the ovarian surface. Histology is useful to differentiate them from a corpus luteum.

Large cysts are characterized by their brown color, lack of vascularization, elongation of the ovarian ligament, and associated lesions. Puncture of the cyst usually leads to diagnosis. Sometimes, however, the fluid is clear and not viscous, in which case cytology is mandatory.

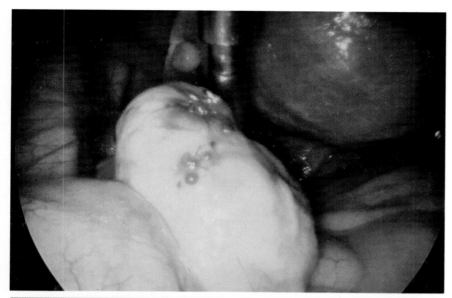

11.8 Superficial implants on the ovarian surface. Note the scarred aspect of the albuginea in front of the forceps.

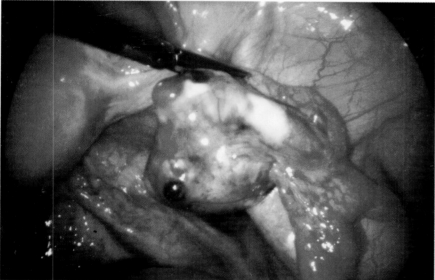

11.9 Ovarian endometriosis. The ovary bears a corpus luteum at its caudal pole. In this case there are deep lesions as well as superficial lesions. A biopsy of the hyperemic lesions generally reveals the presence of ectopic endometrium.

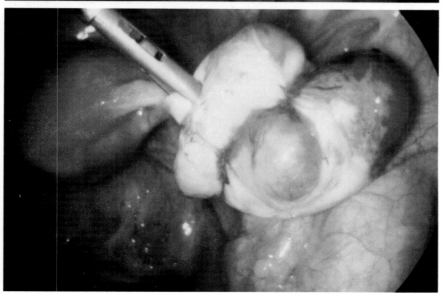

11.10 Endometrioma of the lateral aspect of the ovary, hidden to the observer, unless an ancillary instrument is used.

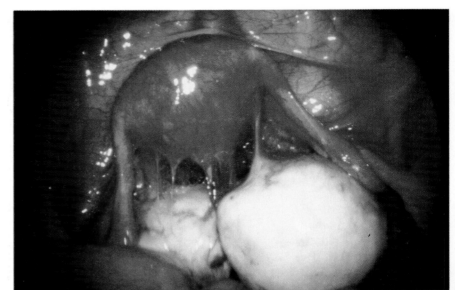

11.11 Ovarian endometrioma, adherent in a typical fashion to the posterior wall of the uterus.

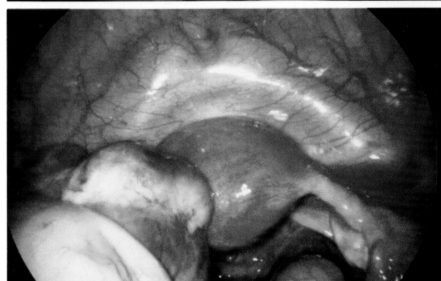

11.12 Endometrioma of the left ovary. Brown discoloration of the cyst wall shining through the ovarian capsule raises the surgeon's suspicion.

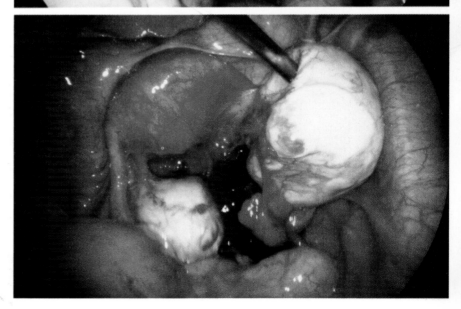

11.13 Endometrioma. Mobilization of the ovary frequently causes the cyst to rupture and spill its contents with the typical "chocolate" appearance.

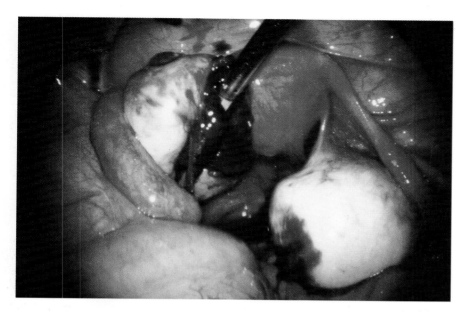

11.14 Identical events on the left side. This sequence of events is common during laparoscopy for endometriosis.

Tubal lesions (Figs. 11.15 through 11.17)

These lesions are rare but need to be detected because their presence changes the surgical approach.

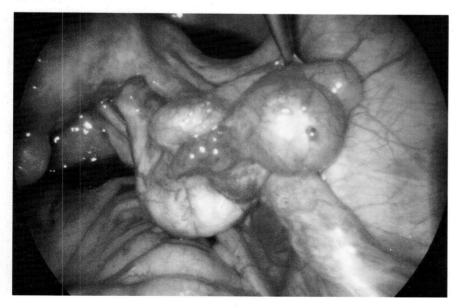

11.15 A more unusual aspect: endometriotic implants are seen on the peritoneal surface of the oviduct. Their presence led to a midampullary phimosis, due to fibrosis.

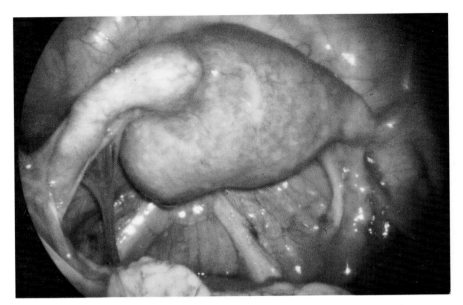

11.16 Typical appearance of salpingitis isthmica nodosa, the etiology of which is still a mystery. Histologically, different lesions can be detected, among them endometriosis.

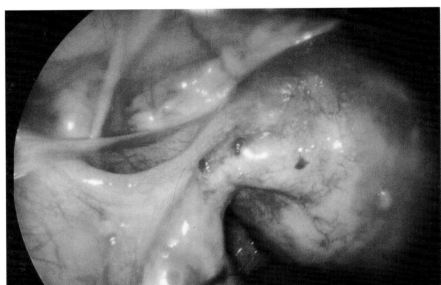

11.17 Endometriotic lesion on the surface of the isthmus of the left tube.

Sampling is mandatory

An effort should be made to biopsy lesions that are thought to be active, especially in the case of ovarian cysts where the cyst wall is not uniformly covered by endometriotic tissue [6, 8]. Peritoneal cytology is of limited value because menstrual reflux probably is the rule rather than the exception [25] and because the result may be negative in the presence of extensive lesions [36]. On the other hand, ovarian cytology is accurate for diagnosis of endometriosis.

Let us not go into a discussion of the difficulties encountered by the pathologist. We shall mention merely that the diagnosis of endometriosis is made only if both glands and stroma are identified.

Laparoscopy is performed not only for diagnosing the presence of the disease but also to determine the extent of the disease accurately. Incomplete diagnosis leads to incomplete treatment; therefore sequelae sometimes appear that are difficult to handle. (Note: Investigations of the gastrointestinal tract such as barium enema and upper GI studies are indicated only when there is clinical suspicion of bowel involvement.)

Diagnostic challenges

They are dual:

– Extensive disease (*frozen pelvis*) because the adhesions are so extensive that often the pelvic cavity cannot be accessed.

– *Burned-out* endometriosis, which may distort the pelvic organs only minimally.

Limits of laparoscopy

The limits are the microscopic lesions [22, 31] and retroperitoneal expansion, in particular at the level of the sacrouterine ligaments and along the course of the ureter.

The existence of microscopic disease, which was suspected on the basis of clinical experience and determination of prostaglandin content in the peritoneal fluid, was confirmed by studies on animals by Schenken [39] and in humans by Murphy [31]. Microscopic disease is probably the initial stage of the disease.

Operative report

Laparoscopy is the main test performed for diagnosis of the disease, and its conclusions will only rarely be challenged. Therefore, the operative report should be as accurate as possible to permit appropriate decisions on the further treatment of the patient. Classifications are essential to allow comparisons between different studies and also to evaluate the effectiveness of a particular treatment regimen.

The AFS classification [2] is the most widely used, as opposed to those of Acosta and Kistner. The AFS classification is reproducible, less biased by the surgeon's subjective "impression," and well quantified; it also distinguishes between bilateral and unilateral lesions. The classification was revised in 1985 [9]. The modifications relate to

– Extent of cul-de-sac obliteration
– Description of adhesions
– Distinction between deep and superficial lesions
– A more detailed description of minimal lesions

The differentiation between severe and extensive lesions disappears, and associated tubal pathology of unrelated origin is evaluated separately.

The changes made in 1985 are of interest but remain to be confirmed. According to Buttram, these modifications should allow for better characterization of the lesions (Table 11.1).

The classifications have the following shortcomings:

– The scoring system—especially the limits between stages—is arbitrary.

– Identical scores in different patients can be due to quite different lesions, probably with different prognoses.

– A particular score can be due to burned-out lesions or active lesions, for which the prognosis is obviously different.

TABLE 11.1 **AFS staging of endometriosis (1985)**

Implants			
Peritoneum	<1 cm	1–3 cm	>3 cm
Superficial	1	2	4
Deep	2	4	6
Right ovary			
Superficial	1	2	4
Deep	4	16	20
Left ovary			
Superficial	1	2	4
Deep	4	16	20
Obliteration of the cul-de-sac: partial, 4; complete, 40			
Adhesions			
Right ovary	<1/3	1/3–2/3	>2/3
Filmy	1	2	4
Dense	4	8	16
Left ovary			
Filmy	1	2	4
Dense	4	8	16
Right tube			
Filmy	1	2	4
Dense	4	8[a]	16
Left tube			
Filmy	1	2	4
Dense	4	8[a]	16

[a] If the infundibulum tubae is involved in the process: 16.

Procedure

General principles

Laparoscopic treatment of endometriosis has two distinct advantages, at least in theory:

– The treatment is performed at the same time as the diagnosis; therefore there is a shorter latency time between treatment and conception than in the case of medical treatment.

– Surgical trauma is less extensive than at laparotomy. This remained a subjective assessment for a long time; however, Fayez [20] has shown that the pregnancy rate in women operated on by means of laparotomy is lower than in women who have undergone laparoscopy. Second-look laparoscopy indicates that all women who have undergone laparotomy have dense adhesions, whereas only 22 % of women operated on by laparoscopy have adhesions, and these are usually filmy in nature and not extremely extensive.

Laparoscopic treatment of endometriosis is difficult because of the nature of this disease.

– An important inflammatory reaction surrounds these lesions, causing changes of the peritoneum and becoming thickened and fibrotic. This can be particularly disturbing close to the ureter. Moreover, this scarring modifies the anatomic relationships between the various organs.

– The invasive behavior of the disease means that

- Retroperitoneal surgery is often required.
- The adhesions generated by the inflammatory process are dense. The serosa disappears secondary to invasion and scarification leads to fusion of the organs. Adhesiolysis is therefore difficult and is contraindicated if the bowel is involved.

Treatment of peritoneal implants

CO_2 laser (Figs. 11.18 through 11.23)

The CO_2 laser is the treatment of choice for these peritoneal lesions. In the form of a defocused beam (500 W/cm^2), the CO_2 laser allows complete destruction with limited unwanted damage to surrounding structures. Once vaporization is completed, the pelvic cavity is copiously rinsed to evacuate the charred debris. Under these circumstances, healing is optimal, no matter how large the treated surface.

In the presence of a deep lesion, one can inject physiologic solution into the retroperitoneal space to loosen the implants from the underlying connective tissue. This is not mandatory if the surgeon has extensive experience with the use of the CO_2 laser. Indeed, the CO_2 laser has the welcome advantage of limiting tissue damage to the treated zone. Therefore, the risk of damage to an underlying structure seems quite low. Some organs, the ureter in particular, can be densely adherent to the peritoneum. Retroperitoneal injection of saline will then create a cleavage plane between ureter and lateral pelvic wall, rather than between ureter and peritoneum.

Other techniques

These are less optimal.

– Monopolar coagulation will cause extensive damage because of the spread of the energy. This effect is amplified by the relatively large contact area of the endoscopic equipment. Tissue destruction is more extensive and the risk of damage to surrounding organs higher. We are convinced that monopolar coagulation ought to be abandoned.

– Bipolar coagulation is precise and satisfactory for superficial lesions. However, the visually observed changes on the surface of a treated lesion do not show whether the depth of destruction is sufficient to encompass the entire lesion. We advise "curetting" the lesions with the jaws of a biopsy forceps to cause small cysts to rupture or peritoneal bridges to collapse.

11.18–11.22 Typical peritoneal implants. The CO_2 laser with a defocused beam is used to destroy the lesion. Note the precision in destruction, both with regard to surface as well as to depth. Carbonized tissue may be removed by means of profuse rinsing.

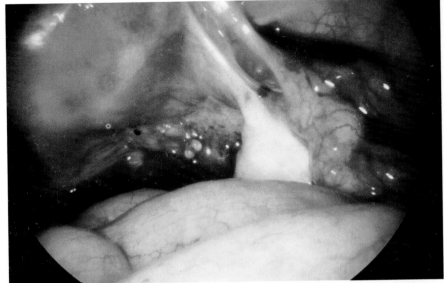

11.18

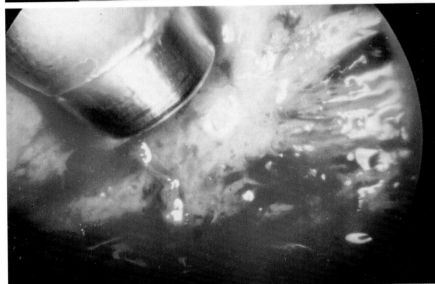

11.19

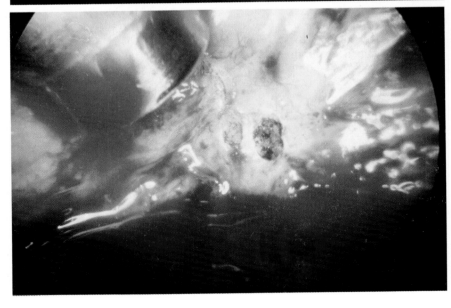

11.20

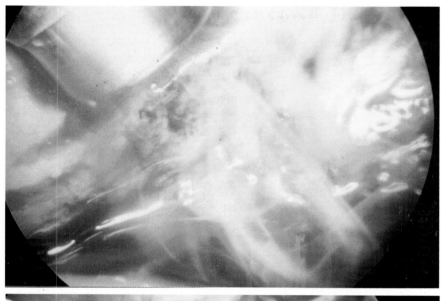

11.21

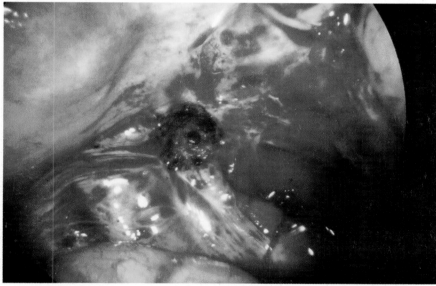

11.22

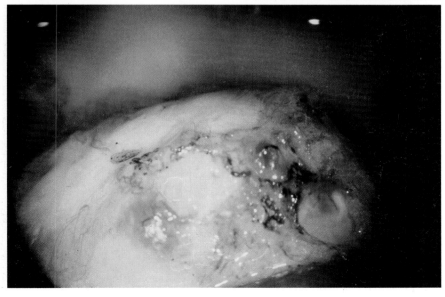

11.23 CO$_2$ laser vaporization of superficial ovarian lesions.

Treatment of ovarian implants

Coagulation of these implants is relatively easy, and monopolar electrocoagulation can also safely be applied. However, to reach lesions on the lateral aspect of the ovary, one has to grasp the ovarian ligament and luxate the ovary upward and laterally by means of a rotating movement.

Treatment of superficial implants should be done with great caution—away from the rectum and ureter. Indeed, superficial lesions respond well to medical treatment, and the risks of surgery are therefore not justified.

Adhesiolysis

The principles of adhesiolysis are described in Chapter 9, which points out that dense adhesions involving the bowel represent a contraindication to laparoscopic surgery. Lysis of dense adhesions is at the outer limit of what is feasible. The CO_2 laser has, in this context, pushed the limits beyond those reached with conventional instruments.

Ovariolysis is usually possible if the ovary is superficially adherent to the uterus or the broad ligament. When it is embedded in the broad ligament, it is beyond the reach of endosurgical lysis.

When salpingolysis is tedious, irreversible damage can be inflicted. One should be prepared to abandon the effort and defer to future microsurgical intervention. At the end of the adhesiolysis, it is possible to cover the raw areas of the pelvic wall and other organs with biodegradable glue to prevent the redevelopment of adhesions. This has, however, not yet been scientifically proven.

Treatment of ovarian cysts

This procedure is independent of the size of the cyst and consists of the following:

Drainage

The cyst is punctured and thoroughly rinsed until the evacuated fluid is clear. One can use a monopolar electrical knife to open large fibrotic endometriomas. The incision is kept small so that the rinsing probe fits snugly into it, so as to avoid spillage. Smaller cysts are drained into the peritoneal cavity or are punctured with a needle.

Drainage only represents incomplete treatment, despite the fact that it enhances medical treatment [25, 28]. Recurrence rates are high when only drainage is accomplished. A cystectomy or destruction of the cyst wall must be performed to prevent recurrence.

Cystectomy

The key to successful cystectomy is finding the cleavage plane, which is not always easy and sometimes causes bleeding. Preventive use of vasopressin is often useful. Otherwise, the procedure is similar to the one described in Chapter 16. When the cyst is large, the procedure can be shortened by excision of the bulging, distended portion of the ovarian capsule.

CO₂ laser vaporization (Fig. 11.24)

The entire lining of the cyst can be destroyed by vaporization, but this is extremely time-consuming. It is advisable to first perform a partial cystectomy. However, vaporization is initiated before profuse bleeding occurs, because this prevents proper use of the CO₂ laser.

When the cyst is small, the endometriotic tissue is usually very active. We therefore advise vaporization of the ovarian stroma once cystectomy—which is difficult—is completed, so as to destroy potential remnants of endometriotic tissue.

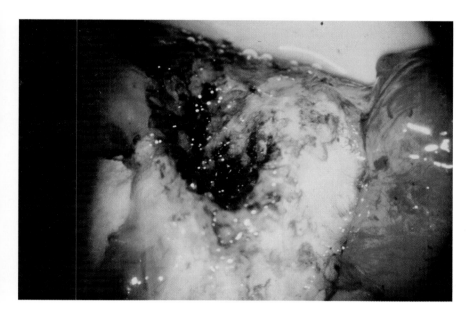

11.24 CO₂ laser vaporization of a small ovarian endometrioma.

Coagulation of the cyst wall

This procedure, with bipolar coagulation, is feasible only for small (2 to 3 cm) cysts, because it is difficult to assess whether the entire cyst lining has been coagulated.

Uterine suspension

There are two indications: treatment of pelvic pain and prevention of recurrence of adhesions at the level of the cul-de-sac. It seems to us that the latter is warranted in severe cases. The technique is described in Chapter 15. The effect of uterine suspension on the success rate of reconstructive surgery is unknown. Acosta [1] ascribes the success of many cases to this intervention. Other series [43] do not confirm this. Our point of view is that the suspension is likely to be valuable if it indeed limits adhesions involving the adnexae.

Laparoscopic uterine nerve ablation (LUNA)

This is a popular procedure in the United States. Its effect on chronic pelvic pain, however, is not well established. Some physicians perform extensive resection of the uterosacral ligaments and rectovaginal septum (*douglasectomy*) for treatment of pain [37]. The value of these extensive procedures needs to be determined.

Surgical strategy

In minimal and mild cases, there is no need for a particular plan. However, a well-defined plan is required for moderate and severe cases, because there is quite often the presence of an ovarian cyst adherent to the posterior leaf of the broad ligament. The objective is to choose the appropriate site for incision of the ovarian cortex while avoiding extensive damage to the ovary.

Our plan is to incise the ovary on the lateral wall rather than puncture and incision of the medial side of the ovary. Indeed, adhesiolysis of the lateral wall from the posterior leaf of the broad ligament quite often causes rupture of the endometriotic cyst. If a previous incision of the medial side of the ovary has been made, a large defect in the ovarian cortex could result. When adhesiolysis is performed first, the site of rupture is also the site for extraction of the cyst. The ovarian defect being on the lateral side, less risk of adhesion formation exists.

When the cul-de-sac is involved, it is advisable to start resecting these lesions, because oozing from operative sites higher up would make the surgery difficult.

Finally, it is foreseeable that endoscopic treatment of severe endometriosis is a long and tedious process, frequently lasting more than $1\frac{1}{2}$ hours. The operating room schedule must be adapted to accommodate that type of operation.

Rules for laparoscopic treatment of endometriosis

To limit recurrence of adhesions after laparoscopic treatment of endometriosis, the following rules must be followed:
- Meticulous hemostasis
- Gentle handling of tissue
- Leave the ovarian cortex with as little damage as possible
- No sutures
- Minimize deperitonealization
- Careful rinsing of the pelvis
- No placement of drains, if possible

With rules and strategy in mind, endoscopic surgery will result in very limited recurrence of adhesions. Laparoscopy does not work miracles; there are always the general rules of reconstructive surgery to be kept in mind.

Results

Between January 1986 and December 1987, we treated 189 patients: 49 (25.9 %) with minimal, 23 (12.2 %) with mild, 63 (33.3 %) with moderate, and 54 (28.6 %) with severe disease. Of the 91 who complained of chronic pelvic pain, 13 were also infertile. In all, 111 patients were treated primarily for infertility (stage I, N = 28; stage II, N = 17; stage III, N = 33; stage IV, N = 33) (Table 11.2). For 61 of the 189 patients (32.3 %) our intervention represented the second round of treatment (Table 11.3).

TABLE 11.2 **Distribution of patient population**

Stage	Minimal	Mild	Moderate	Severe	Total
Number	28	17	33	33	111
Age					
<25	1	0	1	1	3
25–35	23	11	24	23	81
>35	5	6	8	9	28
Duration of infertility					
12–23 months	3	3	5	2	13
24–48 months	17	8	22	21	68
>48 months	8	6	6	10	30
Primary infertility	21	13	24	25	83
Secondary infertility	7	4	9	8	28
Male factor	6	5	6	6	23
Borderline					
spermiogram	4	3	4	4	15
AID	2	2	2	2	8

TABLE 11.3 **Incidence of previous treatment for endometriosis**

	Number	No previous treatment		Previous treatment	
		Number	%	Number	%
Minimal	49	39	79.6	10	20.4
Mild	23	16	69.6	7	30.4
Moderate	63	44	69.8	19	30.2
Severe	54	29	53.7	25	46.3
Total	189	128	67.7	61	32.3

Treatment of severe endometriosis

Among the 54 patients with severe endometriosis, 25 (46.3 %) had been treated previously. The mean AFS score was 72.3 ± 29. Of the 64 endometriomas encountered, 22 were smaller than 3 cm and 42 larger than 3 cm. The technique for removal of these cysts is presented in Table 11.4. The following remarks seem pertinent:

— An ovarian adhesion score of 16 (maximum) occurred in 9 of 10 cases treated by drainage only.

— Cystectomy was possible in 52.4 % of cases if the cyst was larger than 3 cm in diameter but in only 27.3 % if the diameter was less than 3 cm.

— Treatment was complete in 84.1 %.

— Adhesiolysis was complete in 35 (64.8 %) cases with an average adhesion score of 34.8 ± 17 and total score of 63.6 ± 20.9. Adhesiolysis could be only partially completed in 19 cases (35.2 %). The average total score was 85.36 ± 31.26 and the average adhesion score was 58.5 ± 23.54.

TABLE 11.4 **Treatment distribution for deep ovarian endometriosis (stage IV)**
(average AFS score: 72.3 ± 29)

	Number	Drainage			Laser			Cystectomy		
		N	%	Adh. ≥ 16	N	%	Adh. ≥ 16	N	%	Adh. ≥ 16
<3 cm	22	4	18.2	75 %	12	54.5	16.6 %	6	27.2	0
>3 cm	42	6	14.3	100 %	14	33.3	42.8 %	22	52.4	77 %
Total	64	10	15.6	90 %	26	40.6	30.8 %	28	43.6	60.7 %

Pain

Ten patients (11 %) were lost to follow-up. Table 11.5 represents the results obtained after 9 or more months of follow-up. Independent of the stage of the disease, improvement in symptoms occurred in 70 % of cases. Similarly, the recurrence or persistence of pain was of equal proportions among groups.

TABLE 11.5 **Results of pain treatment (author's data)**

	Number	**Improvement, %**	**Cure, %**	**Success, %**	**Failure, %**
Minimal	20	45	35	80	20
Mild	9	55.6	22.2	77.8	22.2
Moderate	31	29	48.4	77.4	22.6
Severe	31	29	42	71	29
Total	91	35.2	40.7	75.8	24.2

Infertility

Of the 111 patients treated because of infertility, 14 were lost to follow-up (12.6 %). Nine other patients were enlisted for in vitro fertilization; 7 of them had extremely severe disease (AFS score >110). The results are given in Table 11.6. The uncorrected pregnancy rate was 40.2 % (35 pregnancies in 87 patients). Cumulative pregnancy rates are presented in Fig. 11.25. Twenty-five (74.2 %) of the 35 pregnancies occurred within 8 months following treatment. No statistically significant difference could be demonstrated between the different stages of the AFS classification.

Results of the treatment in patients with severe endometriosis according to the AFS score are given in Table 11.7. When the total score was >70 or when the adhesion score (including cul-de-sac obliteration) was >50, no pregnancy, either intra- or extrauterine, occurred. However, when the total score was between 41 and 70, the corrected and uncorrected pregnancy rates were, respectively 52.9 % and 58.3 % and thus comparable to those obtained in patients with minimal disease.

TABLE 11.6 **Results of infertility treatment (author's data)**

Stage[a]	**Minimal**		**Mild**		**Moderate**		**Severe**		**Total**	
Results	**N**	**%**	**N**	**%**	**N**	**%**	**N**	**%**	**N**	**%**
N	28		16		33		33		111	
IVF	0		1		4		4		9	
Lost to follow-up	4		1		4		5		14	
Overall results										
N	24		14		25		24		87	
IUP	12	50	4	28.5	10	40	9	37.5	35	40.2
EUP	2	8.3	1	7.1	2	8	0	0	5	5.7
Monthly fec. rate		4.0		1.92		2.98		3.32		3.14
Endosurgery only										
N	18		7		18		19		62	
IUP	11	61	3	42.8	8	44.4	7	36.8	29	46.8
EUP	1	5.5	1	14.2	1	5.5	0	0	3	4.8

[a] There was no statistically significant difference between stages.

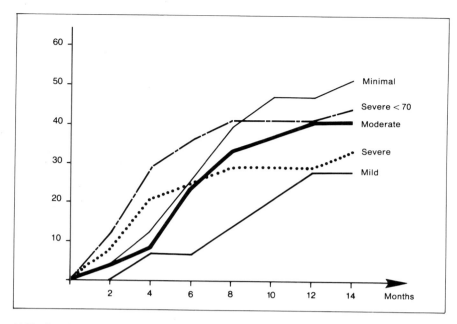

11.25 Cumulative pregnancy rates.

TABLE 11.7 **Stage IV—fertility outcome as a function of the AFS score**

	AFS score	≤70	>70
N		17	7
IUP		9	0
%		52.9[a]	0[a]
	Adhesions	**≤50**	**>50**
N		17	7
IUP		9	0
%		52.9[a]	0[a]
	Implants	**≤20**	**>20**
N		8	16
IUP		6	3
%		75[b]	18.6[b]

[a] χ^2 (Yates) = 3.88; $p = 0.018$.
[b] χ^2 (Yates) = 5.00; $p = 0.011$.

Discussion

Multiple studies have been published showing that laparoscopic treatment is at least as effective as the medical treatment modalities in the minimal and mild stages. The data of the main publications are given in Table 11.8. The majority of authors agree that laparoscopy is unnecessary in these groups. However, laparoscopy has the definite advantage of offering treatment at the time of diagnosis, reducing the latency period between diagnosis and pregnancy. Although the value of endoscopic surgery still has to be compared to no treatment, the minimal invasiveness and almost complete absence of risks seem to warrant laparoscopic destruction or removal of the endometriotic tissue. For stages III and IV, surgery is required. Adhesions simply do not disappear with medical treatment. Moreover, several studies have shown that treatment of

TABLE 11.8 **Fertility outcome after CO_2 laser endosurgery (% pregnant, uncorrected)**

Author	Total		Mild		Moderate		Severe	
	N	% Preg.	N	% Preg.	N	% Preg.	N	% Preg.
Feste [21]	140	82 (59 %)	106	62 (58 %)	31	18 (58 %)	3	2 (67 %)
Daniell [14]	48	34 (54 %)	24	16 (67 %)	15	7 (47 %)	9	3 (33 %)
Davis [15]	64	37 (58 %)	31	20 (65 %)	26	15 (58 %)	7	2 (29 %)
Martin [29]	115	54 (47 %)	56	23 (41 %)	45	22 (49 %)	14	9 (64 %)
Nehzat [33]	102	62 (61 %)	24	18 (75 %)	51	32 (63 %)	27	15 (56 %)
Paulsen [35]	282	150 (53 %)	170	97 (57 %)	112	53 (47 %)	0	
Total	851	472 (55 %)	483	278 (58 %)	304	156 (51 %)	64	33 (52 %)

cystic endometriosis of the ovary is not feasible with medication only [10, 19], which is not surprising, because the cyst consists of fibrous material, similar to adhesions [8]. The real question is whether laparoscopic treatment is possible in the later stages, especially in stage IV. Our results indicate that ovarian lesions can be dealt with in 84 % of cases and adhesions can be completely removed in 65 % of cases. The main difficulty, therefore, seems to be the treatment of adhesions. Looking at treatment of ovarian cysts (Table 11.4), one can see that the cysts that could only be drained involved ovaries with a maximal adhesion score. This confirms that the adhesions are the main problem, preventing appropriate surgical treatment of the lesion.

When the total AFS score is > 70, no pregnancy occurred. The same is seen with an adhesion score > 50. Detailed analysis indicates that the bulk of the score is due to the adhesions. The limit of laparoscopic surgery therefore depends on the extent of the adhesions more than on the extent of the endometriosis itself.

Would a microsurgical intervention be more successful? We would answer that question as follows:

– For stage II, the results of laparoscopic surgery are similar to those obtained by microsurgery [23, 24] (Table 11.9). Comparison is difficult, due to use of different staging systems, but the proportion of patients in the class of severe lesions is similar in all three systems.

– When a tubal score is calculated according to the French system of staging tubal disease, these patients would all fall under the category labeled *severe*. It has been clearly demonstrated that the results of microsurgery are poor in those cases and that it is better to advise IVF for those patients [27]. The number of patients with a total AFS score of > 70 is limited in our series, unfortunately. Other series will have to confirm the extremely poor outcome in these patients. However, we would like to see stage V implemented in the AFS classification, to indicate a highly unfavorable prognosis after surgical intervention.

TABLE 11.9 **Comparative results of microsurgery**

	Moderate		Severe	
	Number	**%**	**Number**	**%**
Gordts	99	42.4	57	35.1
Olive	43	51.2	34	29.4
Current study	25	40	24	37.5

These patients should be treated by IVF, although surgery may be indicated to liberate the ovaries as much as possible in order to improve ovulation. The reduced trauma, followed by fewer adhesions, is the main advantage of laparoscopic surgery. However, no study has ever clearly demonstrated this fundamental statement. There is only the retrospective study from Fayez [20], who compared the fertility outcome between patients operated on by microsurgery and those operated on by laparoscopy. He concluded that the better outcome following laparoscopy was due to a difference in adhesion formation.

Recurrence of adhesions after laparoscopic adhesiolysis is, however, common. Indeed, partial recurrence occurred in 7 out of 17 (49 %) adnexae after complete adhesiolysis. Improvement of the adhesion score occurred in only 5 of 14 cases (35.7 %) after incomplete adhesiolysis. On the other hand, we have never observed a worsening of the adhesion score. Therefore, we consider laparoscopic treatment to be an ideal approach but believe that it should follow the rules of tubal microsurgery: gentle tissue handling, minimal trauma to the ovary, good hemostasis, and probably also a second-look laparoscopy.

Indications

Patients with endometriosis should be divided into two groups:
 – Minimal and mild lesions, in which cases laparoscopic treatment is always possible, even without sophisticated equipment.
 – Moderate and severe lesions, where complete treatment is more difficult and sometimes even impossible. It seems to us that these cases should be treated by experienced surgeons with access to sophisticated equipment, such as a CO_2 laser.

The value of laparoscopy in assessing therapeutic efficacy and in long-term follow-up

Assessment of success rates

After surgical treatment

Second-look laparoscopy after microsurgery for severe endometriosis is justifiable because:
  - The operation is usually a long one.
  - The adhesiolysis is usually difficult and bloody.

This reasoning is confirmed through observation by Brossens [7], who, in 1981, suggested two successive laparotomies for the treatment of severe cases and by Schenken, who reported a high incidence of adhesions in patients undergoing second-look laparoscopy. Our experience in patients after laparotomy for laser treatment of endometriosis confirmsthese statements. Second-look laparoscopy in our department is performed approximately 2 months after the treatment. We consider this time lapse to be sufficient for postoperative healing but soon enough that adhesiolysis is easy to perform at that time.

After medical treatment

Second-look laparoscopy is not systematically performed, certainly not after treatment of minimal or mild stages, especially in women over 35 and without further desire for fertility. On the other hand, in the presence of moderate or severe lesions in patients with infertility, second-look laparoscopy seems indicated because:
  - It will detect residual disease in the severe cases and possibly complete treatment.
  - Dmowski [18] has indicated that adhesions can appear on implants during medical treatment. These adhesions could be the result of a delay in suppression of the implants by the drugs. This needs to be confirmed.
  - The ectopic endometrium contains hormone receptors in cytosol [4, 26, 44] and nucleus [24], but in smaller quantities than the eutopic endometrium [33]; therefore hormonal regulation is disturbed [45]. Schweppe [41] has demonstrated that the efficiency of medical treatment is correlated with the degree of differentiation of the ectopic endometrium.
  - Finally, studies on residual lesions after medical treatment (with danazol) have shown that endometrial tissue is demonstrated in 15 % of cases, showing viable cells. This probably explains the recurrence after medical treatment [42].

In conclusion, second-look laparoscopy seems to be necesssary to evaluate a medical treatment regimen.

Long-term follow-up

Recurrence [3, 16, 46]

Recurrence seems to correlate with the initial stage of the disease, the occurrence of pregnancy soon after treatment, and the treatment modality. Figures vary around 30 % [3, 17]. Recurrence remains a vague concept. Indeed, few studies encompass a detailed anatomic description allowing differentiation between the persistence of existing lesions or the appearance of new lesions. Moreover, the absence of correlation between symptoms and findings was well demonstrated by Williams and Schenken [46, 40]. The sequelae of endometriosis can mimic the symptoms of endometriosis, falsely indicating the persistence of disease.

Treatment failure

Whether one deals with persistent pain or infertility, laparoscopy plays an important role. However, when dealing with chronic pelvic pain, one should refrain from repetitive laparoscopies, especially if a previous endoscopic examination was negative. When dealing with infertility, the situation is different because it is difficult to extend medical treatment beyond several months. It is also possible to combine a second laparoscopic evaluation with ovarian stimulation—for assisted reproductive purposes—in cases of minimal, mild, and moderate extent of the disease. When dealing with severe cases, ovarian stimulation is done only when no ovarian cysts are present.

References

1. Acosta A., Buttram V.C., Besch P.K., Malinak L.R., Franklin R.R., Vanderheyen J.P., « A proposed classification of pelvic endometriosis », *Obstet. Gynecol.*, 1973; 12 : 49.
2. The American Fertility Society, « Classification of endometriosis », *Fertil. Steril.*, 1979; 32 : 633.
3. Barbieri R.L., Evans S., Kistner R.W., « Danazol in the treatment of endometriosis. Analysis of 100 cases with a four year follow-up », *Fertil. Steril.*, 1982; 37 : 737.
4. Bergquist A., Nillius S.S., Wide L., Lindgren A., « Estrogen and progesterone receptors concentration in endometriotic tissue and intrauterine endometrium », *Acta Obstet. Gynecol. Scand.*, suppl., 1981; 101 : 53-58.
5. Biberoglu K.O., Behrman S.J., « Dosage respect of Danazol therapy in endometriosis : short term and long term effectiveness », *Am. J. Obstet. Gynecol.*, 1981; 139 : 645.
6. Blaustein A., « Pelvic endometriosis, in pathology of the female genital tract », 2nd ed., Springer Verlag, Berlin, 1982.
7. Brossens I., Koninckx P.R., Boeckx W., « Endometriosis », *Clin. Obstet. Gynaecol.*, 1981; 8 : 639.
8. De Brux J., « Histopathologie gynécologique », 2e édition, Masson, Paris, 1981.
9. Buttram V.C., « Evolution of the revised American Fertility Society classification of endometriosis », *Fertil. Steril.*, 1985; 43 : 347.
10. Buttram V.C., Reiter R.C., Ward S., « Treatment of endometriosis with Danazol. Report of 6 years prospective Study », *Fertil. Steril.*, 1985; 3 : 533.
11. Buttram V.C., Belue J.L., Reiter R., « Interim report of a study of Danazol for the treatment of endometriosis », *Fertil. Steril.*, 1982; 37 : 478.
12. Chany Y., « Endométriome ovarien. Etude bibliographique et statistique », Thèse de médecine, Clermont-Ferrand, 1984.
13. Cornelie P., Brossens I., « Morphologic evaluation of pelvic endometriosis in endometriosis », 1st International Symposium, Clermont-Ferrand, 1986.
14. Daniell J.F., « Basic and advanced, laser surgery in gynecology », Treatment of gynecology tumors, 1985, 345-356. Ed. Appleton Century Crofts, Connecticut.
15. Davis G.D., « Management of endometriosis and its associated adhesions with the CO_2 laser laparoscope », *Obstet. Gynecol.*, 1986; 68 : 422.
16. Dmowski W.P., Cohen M.R., « Antigonadotropin (Danazol) in the treatment of endometriosis. Evaluation of post treatment fertility and three year follow-up data », *Am. J. Obstet. Gynecol.*, 1978; 41 : 130.
17. Dmowski W.P., « Danazol in the treatment of endometriosis and infertility »; *Prog. Clin. Biol. Res.* 1982; 112 : 167.

18. Dmowski W.P., Cohen M.R., « Treatment of endometriosis with an antigo-nadotropin : Danazol : a laparoscopic and histologic evaluation », *Obstet. Gynecol.*, 1975; 46 : 147.

19. Donnez J., « CO_2 laser laparoscopy in infertile women with endometriosis and women with adnexal adhesions », *Fertil. Steril.*, 1987; 48 : 390.

20. Fayez J.A., Collazo L., « Comparison of laparotomy and laparoscopy in the treatment of moderate and severe stages of endometriosis », AFS meeting abst 317, 1986.

21. Feste J.R., « Endoscopic laser surgery in gynecology ». In : Reproductive surgery, Post-graduate Course Syllabus, American Fertility Society, Chicago, 1985, 51-69.

22. Goldstein D., Decholnoky C., Emans S., « Adolescent endometriosis », *J. Adolesc. Health Care*, 1980; 1 : 37.

23. Gordts S., Boeckx W., Brossens I., « Microsurgery of endometriosis in infertile patients », *Fertil. Steril.*, 1984; 42 : 520.

24. Gould S.F., Shannon J.M., Cunha G.R., « Nuclear estrogen bindings sites in human endometriosis », *Fertil. Steril.*, 1983; 39 : 520.

25. Halme J., Hammond M.G., Mulka J.F., Ras S.G., Talbert L.M., « Retrograde menstrua-tion in healthy women and in patient with endometriosis », *Obstet. Gynecol.*, 1984; 64 : 151.

26. Janne O., Kauppila A., Kotto E., Lantto T., Rohnberg L., Vihko R., « Estrogen and progestin receptors in endometriosis lesions : comparison with endometrial tissue », *Am. J. Obstet. Gynecol.*, 1981; 141 : 562.

27. Mage G., Bruhat M.A., Bouquet J., Canis M., Chabrand S., Dellenbach P., Dubuisson J.B., Henri-Suchet J., Madelenat P., Mintz M., Pouly J.L., Salat-Baroux J., « Score d'opérabilité tubaire » 23e Assises Françaises de Gynécologie, Poitiers, 1987.

28. Manhes H., Mage G., Pouly J.L., Bruhat M.A., « Technique et résultats du traitement cœlioscopique de l'endométriome ovarien : à propos de 30 cas », *Gynécologie*, 1980; 31 : 149.

29. Martin D.C., « Operative laparoscopy with the carbon dioxide laser for the treatment of endometriosis associated with infertility », *J. Reprod Med.*, 1986; 31 : 1089.

30. Mondie F., « Endométriose et cœlioscopie », Thèse de médecine, Clermont-Ferrand, 1982.

31. Murphy A., Green W., Bobbie D., de la Cruz Z., Rock J., « Unsuspected endometriosis documented by scanning electron microscopy in visually normal peritoneum », *Fert. Steril.*, 1986; 46 : 522-524.

32. Nagata Y., Nakamura G., Kusuda M., « Therapeutic effect and side effect of Danazol in endometriosis », *Asia Oceania J. Obstet. Gynecol.*, 1982; 8 : 229.

33. Nehzat C., Crowgey S.R., « Surgical treatment of endometriosis via laser laparoscopy », *Fertil. Steril.*, 1986; 45 : 778.

34. Olive D.L., Martin D.C., « Treatment of endometriosis-associated infertility with CO_2 laser laparoscopy : the use of one- and two-parameter exponential models », *Fertil. Steril.*, 1987; 48 : 18.

35. Paulsen J.D., Asmar P., « Analysis of the first 150 pregnancies after laser laparoscopy », presented at the ASCCP/GLS Meeting, Boston, 1986.

36. Portuondo J.A., Herran C., Echanojauregui A.D., Riego A.G., « Peritoneal flushing and biopsy in laparoscopically diagnosed endometriosis », *Fertil. Steril.*, 1982; 38 : 538.

37. Reich H., Martin D.C. (A paraître), *Fertil. Steril.*

38. Rock J.A., Guzick D.S., Sengos C., Schweditsch M., Sapp K.C., Jones H.W., « The conservative surgical treatment of endometriosis : evaluation of pregnancy success with respect to the extent of disease as categorized using contemporary classification systems », *Fertil. Steril.*, 1981; 35 : 131.

39. Schencken R.S., Asch R.H., Williams R.F., Hodgen G.A., « Etiology of infertility in monkeys with endometriosis : luteinized unruptured follicles, luteal phase defects, pelvic adhesions, and spontaneous abortions », *Fertil. Steril.*, 1984; 41 : 22.

40. Schencken R.S., Malinak L.R., « Reoperation after initial treatment of endometriosis with conservative surgery », *Am. J. Obstet. Gynecol.*, 1978; 131 : 406.

41. Schweppe K.W., Wynn R.M., « Endocrine dependency of endometriosis on ultrastruc-tural study », *Eur. J. Obstet. Gynecol. Reprod. Biol.*, 1984; 17 : 193.

42. Schweppe K.W., Dmowsky W.P., Wynn R.M., « Ultrastructural change in endometriotic tissue during danazol therapy », *Fertil. Steril.*, 1981; 20 : 36.

43. Spangler D.B., Jones G., Jones H.W., « Infertility due to endometriosis. Conservative surgical therapy », *Am. J. Obstet. Gynecol.*, 1971; 109 : 850.

44. Tamaya T., Motoyama T., Ohono Y., Ide N., Tsurusaki T., Okada H., « Steroid receptors level and histology of adenomyosis and endometriosis », *Fertil. Steril.*, 1979; 31 : 396.

45. Vierikko P., Kauppila A., Isomaa V., Ronnberg L., Vihko R., « Effect of gestrinome in endometriosis tissue and endometrium », *Fertil. Steril.*, 1985.

46. Williams T.J., Pratt J.H., « Endometriosis in 1000 consecutive coeliotomies, incidence and management », *Am. J. Obstet Gynecol.*, 1977; 120 : 245.

12

Extrauterine pregnancy

Improved diagnosis of extrauterine pregnancy—via subunit hCG titers and ultrasonography—and refinements in laparoscopic operative techniques led us to begin laparoscopic treatment of this condition in 1974 [1]. Continued improvements in instrumentation and operative technique have resulted in laparoscopy being well established and safe for this purpose [11], with excellent conservation of fertility potential [18].

Radical treatment (i.e., salpingectomy) is performed when no further fertility is desired or when the risk of recurrence of ectopic pregnancy is considered too high.

Introduction

The incidence of ectopic pregnancy is on the rise in all developed countries. In France, the rate was 1 ectopic pregnancy per 131 deliveries in 1975; by 1981, it had risen to 1 ectopic pregnancy per 76 deliveries [4]. Similarly, in the United States [3], the number of extrauterine pregnancies tripled between 1967 and 1976. According to Weström, this rise is due to the increased incidence of sexually transmitted diseases [32].

The development of more accurate ultrasonography and more sensitive hCG tests has allowed earlier diagnosis of ectopic pregnancy and reduced the incidence of negative laparoscopy. However, the most accurate diagnostic technique is still direct visualization via laparoscopy. Table 12.1 presents our plan for differential diagnosis of ectopic pregnancy versus abortion. This differential diagnosis is still difficult in the early stages, and it may sometimes be helpful to perform frozen sections of the curettings in search for villi if one wants to avoid laparoscopy. Early diagnosis permits a more conservative surgical approach.

On the other hand, new techniques of assisted reproductive technology, the possibility of radical endosurgical treatment, and detailed analysis of the results obtained with conservative surgery have led to a more critical evaluation of the indications for conservative surgery. One should consider the following parameters:
- History
- The appearance of the ectopic pregnancy
- The appearance of the contralateral tube
- Age and family planning method(s) of the patient

We first describe the procedure and then evaluate the indications.

TABLE 12.1 **Differential diagnosis of ectopic pregnancy**

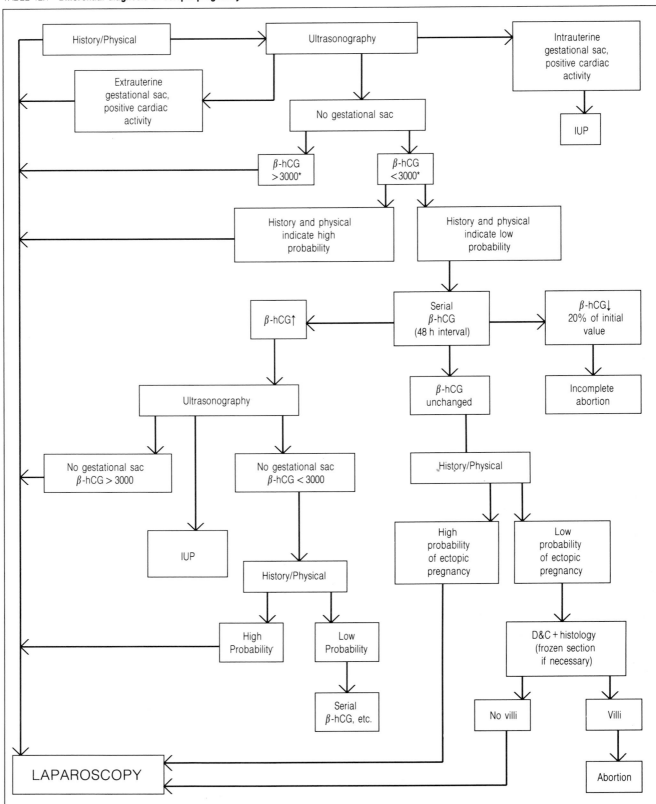

* The absolute number used as the "break-off point" depends on the sensitivity of the test used. The number should correspond to the mean hCG level of a normal pregnancy at 6 weeks (post menses).

Procedure

Preparation

Two suprapubic trocars are inserted, one for the introduction of a forceps and the other for the rinsing-aspiration probe (Triton). Positioning of the trocars depends on the site of implantation of the ectopic pregnancy and on the preference of the surgeon. Usually, the Triton is inserted at the site contralateral to the pregnancy. Some surgeons prefer the instrument to be on the left no matter where the pregancy is located.

Conservative treatment (Figs. 12.1 through 12.9)

Step 1

The first step is aspiration and evacuation of blood and clots, followed by rinsing. Next, the operator locates the pregnancy and evaluates whether an endosurgical approach is feasible.

Step 2

The second step is chemical hemostasis. The principle is to induce vasoconstriction of the vascular bed supplying the ectopic pregnancy. Diluted Ornipressin (POR 8 Sandoz, 5 mlU in 20 mL physiologic saline) is injected into the mesosalpinx. A 19-gauge spinal needle is used percutaneously. The injection must be strictly extravascular, causing immediate distention of the mesosalpinx over its entire length. Injection can be made just beneath the conceptus or further away with identical effect. Within a minute, the entire tube blanches.

Step 3

The third step is the salpingotomy, performed at the antemesenterial border of the inner third of the hematosalpinx, which is the site of implantation of the conceptus. The unipolar needle of the Triton is used in the cutting mode to open the tube over 1 to 2 cm. This is usually bloodless and one can see the blood clots and villi emerge from the tubal lumen.

Step 4

The fourth step is extraction of the products of conception. The rinsing probe is inserted into the incision and aspiration started. This will generally be sufficient to evacuate the pregnancy; occasionally, injection of fluid under high pressure helps break up the blood clots. Three difficulties may arise:

– Extraction is easy, but the clots do not pass into the rinsing probe. These clots are then ejected into the cul-de-sac to break them up before reaspiration.

– The villi do not evacuate easily. A grasping forceps is introduced into the lumen and the pregnancy gently teased out of the tube without damaging the mucosa.

– The blood clots clog the Triton. The instrument can be cleared by connecting—outside the abdomen—the aspirator to the distal end of the probe.

The incision into the tube is left unclosed.

Step 5

The fifth step is assessment of tubal status:

– Assure that the affected tube is truly empty. Spreading apart the edges of the incision with a forceps permits visual inspection of the lumen for detecting residual trophoblast, which is typically bright white.

– Evaluate further fertility chances by inspecting the contralateral tube.

Step 6

The sixth step is the thorough lavage of the pelvic cavity, alternately rinsing and aspirating a physiologic solution—an easily performed maneuver with an apparatus such as the Triton. To avoid having the bowel stick to the aspiration cannula, it is a good idea to hold the bowel away with a forceps. The tip of the probe is held constantly under water to avoid aspirating excessive amounts of CO_2 gas. Even if the operator is careful to observe this precaution, a high-flow insufflator comes in handy at this point to replace rapidly lost gas. The Trendelenburg position is progressively reversed to evacuate fluid that has accumulated higher in the abdominal cavity.

Step 7

The seventh step is the immediate postoperative period:

– Drainage of the peritoneal cavity is generally unnecessary, but a drain may be installed for 12 to 48 h. It is used for evacuation of residual fluid rather than for the detection of hemorrhage. A drain of the Jackson-Pratt type is inserted through a suprapubic trocar without flap valve.

– Postoperative recovery is reduced to 2 or 3 days. (Note from translator: The hospital stay in European countries is, on the average, three to four times longer than in the United States. It is not unusual, in Europe, for a patient who has undergone laparotomy for ectopic pregnancy to remain in the hospital for 6 to 8 days.) Fall in β-hCG titers is closely monitored. Postoperative treatment with corticosteroids and tetracycline is prescribed when adhesiolysis was performed simultaneously on the contralateral tube. In all other cases, no medical treatment is required.

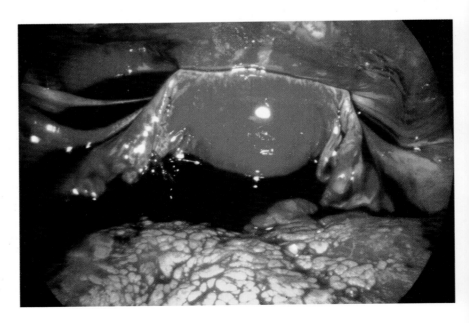

12.1 Hemoperitoneum due to an ectopic pregnancy.

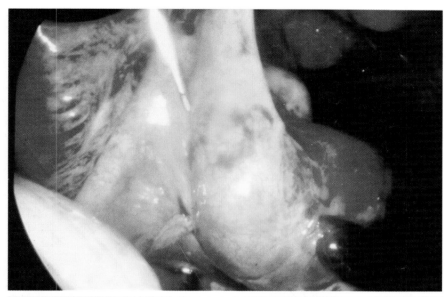

12.2 The pregnancy is located as soon as the hemoperitoneum is evacuated. Ornipressin (a vaso-pressin derivative) is injected into the mesosalpinx.

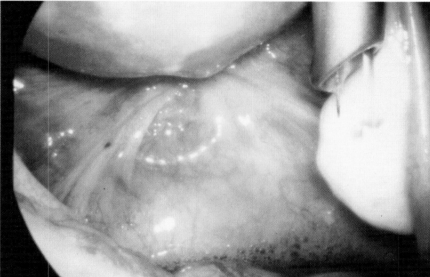

12.3 The Triton is inserted. One can see its trifold action: rinsing, aspiration, and cutting with a monopolar needle electrode.

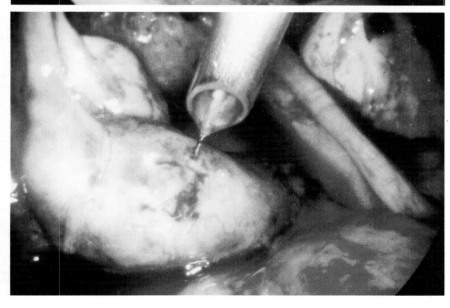

12.4 and 12.5 Incision of the tubal wall at the proximal part of the hematosalpinx. Note the blanching of tissue due to injection of ornipressin, as compared to Fig. 12.2.

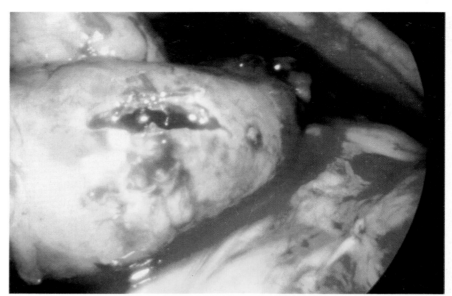

12.5   The incision is made.

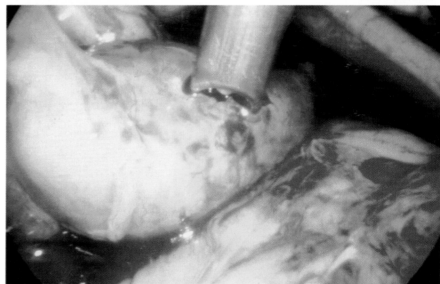

12.6   The tubal contents are aspirated.

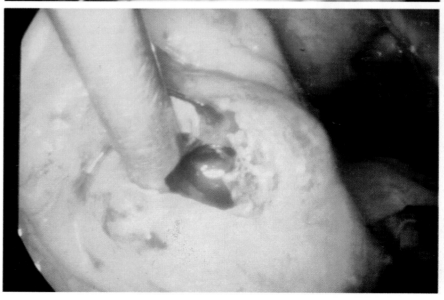

12.7   The tubal lumen is visually inspected.

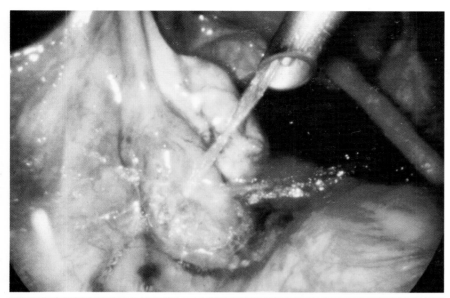

12.8 Rinsing-aspiration of the peritoneal cavity.

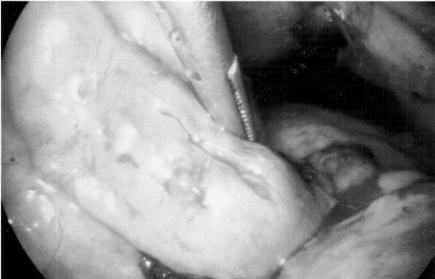

12.9 Appearance of the incision at the end of the procedure.

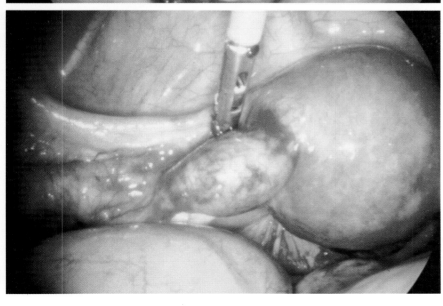

12.10 Isthmic ectopic pregnancy.

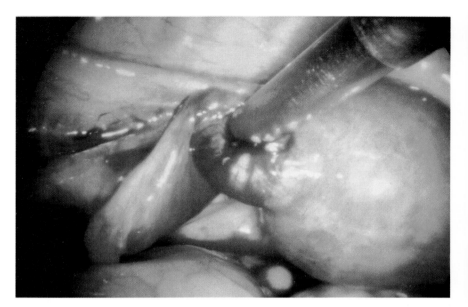

12.11 Aspiration of the contents after injection of ornipressin and incision of the wall.

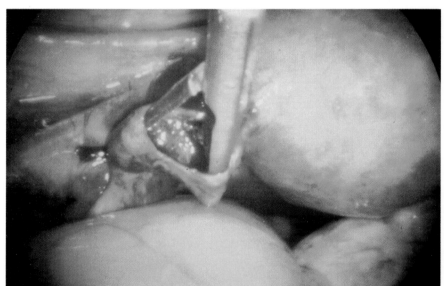

12.12 The tubal lumen is visually inspected.

General comments

The current technique has evolved considerably over the years. Early on, we attempted to abort the pregnancy through the fimbriated end of the tube. Then, from 1974 to 1978, we introduced salpingotomy with monopolar cutting current and evacuation of the tubal contents using a Karman cannula. Hemostasis was obtained by compression with forceps. In 1978, we developed the Triton, which greatly simplified incision and aspiration. Finally, introduction of synthetic vasopressin (POR 8) resolved the biggest problem: obtaining hemostasis. To date, we have performed over 500 cases.

Specialized instrumentation

The Triton was designed for treatment of ectopic pregnancy. It is a multifunctional apparatus, requiring some training to optimize coordination of the different functions: rinsing and exit of the needle are hand-controlled, whereas aspiration and current activation are foot-controlled. A great advantage of the instrument is that it eliminates frequent exchange of instruments.

Without the Triton or a similar instrument, it is difficult to perform the procedure. The Triton has the largest diameter of all instruments for suction/rinsing available at this time. An improved version of the instrument is currently being developed: the Polytron (Synergy; Vichy, France).

Mandatory salpingotomy (Figs. 12.13, 12.14, 12.15)

Salpingotomy is required in all cases involving hematosalpinx. It is tempting, especially when the pregnancy protrudes partially through the fimbriated end, to omit the incision. This is what we did initially. Several cases of persisting ectopic pregnancy occurred because villi remained in the tube. Only when the pregnancy is implanted on the fimbriated end itself can one bypass making the incision. Also, the incision should be made proximal to the uterus, where the conceptus itself is actually implanted. The distal part of the hematosalpinx contains only blood clots.

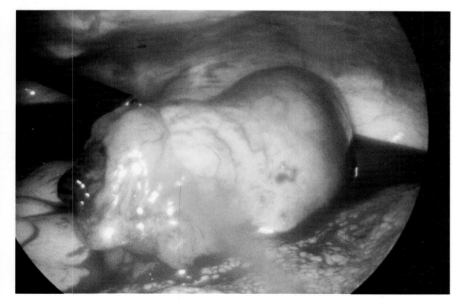

12.13 and 12.14 Distal ampullary ectopic pregnancy.

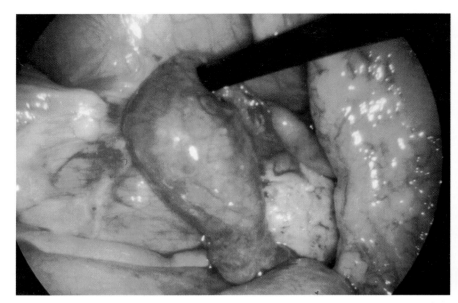

12.14 Distal ampullary ectopic pregnancy.

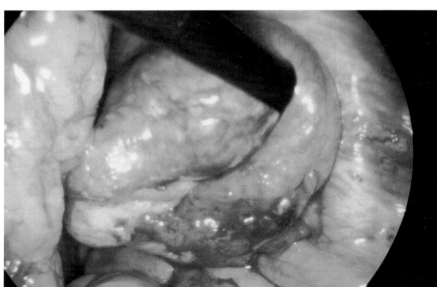

12.15 Situs after surgical treatment, which included a salpingotomy, in order to avoid persistent trophoblast.

The importance of hemostasis

Hemostasis is the most difficult aspect of conservative surgical management of tubal pregnancy. Some bleeding occurs at the incision site but even more from the placental bed. At laparotomy, hemostasis is obtained by closing the incision, coagulation of the placental bed, or ligation of vessels in the mesosalpinx. These manipulations are traumatizing, however. Vasopressin is a potent vasoconstrictor, arresting bleeding quickly. The effect lasts approximately 2 h, during which natural clotting of vessels occurs, so that there is no bleeding when the effects of the drug wear off. We have experienced only one case of hemorrhage, 4 h following vasopressin, in a patient treated with anticoagulants. Of special note: it is imperative that the injection of vasopressin be extravascular. Accidental intravascular injection could cause a major cardiovascular accident. Occasionally, bradycardia or transient hypertension can be observed even when the drug is used correctly. In over 250 cases, only one complication occurred: in an anemic patient presenting acute pulmonary edema 6 h after use of the drug. The cause-effect relationship in this case is still not clear to us.

Vasopressin is used to prevent bleeding. It permits surgery under optimal, bloodless conditions. It also seems that, with it, the products of conception are easier to remove. Use of vasopressin does not affect subsequent tubal function. The incision heals well, as we have observed at second-look laparoscopy. Fertility is not affected. In 54 patients who underwent surgery without POR 8, 61.1 % experienced subsequent intrauterine pregnancy and 22.2 % a recurrent ectopic pregnancy. With the use of POR 8, on the other hand, these rates were 67.4 % and 13.7 %, respectively. There is no statistically significant difference (Table 12.2).

TABLE 12.2 **Fertility outcome in relation to vasopressin use, site of pregnancy and tubal rupture**

	Number	IUP		EUP	
		Number	%	Number	%
Hemostasis					
With vasopressin	169	116	68.6	15	8.9
Without vasopressin	54	33	61.1	12	22.2
Tubal rupture					
Yes	62	39	62.9	9	14.5
No	161	100	64.6	18	11.2
Site of pregnancy					
Isthmus	48	29[a,b]	60.4	9	18.3
Ampulla	151	93[a,c]	61.2	17	11.2
Infundibulum	19	16[b,c]	84.2	1	5.3

[a] = NS.
[b,c] $p < 0.05$ (χ^2 test).
Note: All other comparisons not statistically significant.

Radical treatment

The first four steps are the same as the first four steps outlined previously. Thereafter, the isthmus tubae is coagulated at ± 1 cm from the uterine horn and transected. The Triton is used to "aspirate" the distal stump. This maneuver stabilizes the tube. Next, the mesosalpinx is alternately coagulated and transected. The tube is extracted through the trocar in which the Triton was inserted. Emptying the tube prior to removal is not necessary but usually required in order to permit easier removal. We advise doing this prior to the salpingectomy. Next, a Filshie clip is placed on the proximal stump for prevention of recurrence of an ectopic pregnancy in the stump. (Note from translator: Filshie clips are not approved for use in the United States as of this writing.)

Semm [26] described a technique of salpingectomy using endothermia instead of bipolar coagulation. A study on 100 patients was published by Dubuisson [8], who describes this technique well.

Results of conservative treatment (503 cases)

Failure of the procedure

Incomplete removal (i.e., persistent ectopic pregnancy) occurred in 21 cases (4.2 %). Of these, 11 required laparotomy and 10 were treated with a second laparoscopy. One case was revealed to be a tubal chorioepithelioma. This relatively high failure rate might lead one to reject the method out of hand. However, let us keep in mind that these are results of a newly developed technique that is bound to undergo some "childhood diseases."

Let us analyze these figures. Of the failures, 11 were due to inexperience of the operator, 5 to faulty technique (aspiration through the fimbriated end), and 6 to nonobservance of the contraindications. Therefore 11 failures should, in fact, have been avoided. The main reason—inexperience of the operator—will likely persist, because in a university hospital residents are undergoing the process of training. Therefore the true incidence of failure in experienced hands is estimated to be approximately 2 %.

Clinical course of failures

Failures typically present as chronic ectopic pregnancies with the formation of a hematocele within 10 to 20 days following the first intervention. We advocate repetitive measurement of β-hCG titers until they are negative to assure complete removal of the trophoblast. We measured β-hCG in 69 successive cases and compared the results to values of 7 failures previously recorded [23]. When surgery has been successful, the decrease is rapid during the first 48 h (initially the half-life of hCG is 19.4 h). Later, the rate of decay is slower (with a half-life of 63.9 h). These relative values are not dependent on the initial absolute value of β-hCG. In case of failure, the decay of the hCG titer is slower. At day 2 or 3 postoperatively, the concentration (in percent) was higher than the mean (of the entire group) ± 2 SD except for one case, where it was higher than the mean ± 1 SD. However, at days 8 and 7, the latter case showed a titer higher than the mean ± 2 SD. These data are highly significant.

A β-hCG titer at day 2 or 3 postintervention permits prediction of the outcome, as shown in Table 12.3:

– Success is assured if the titer at 48 h is less than or equal to 15 % of the initial value, obtained the day of surgery.

– Failure is likely if the titer is higher than 35 % of the initial value.

– For values in between those above, the titers must be followed until total clearance occurs.

Prevention of failures

Three principal aspects are to be noted:

– Salpingostomy is mandatory in all cases of hematosalpinx. Aspiration through the fimbriated end should be abandoned.

– This intervention should be done by experienced laparoscopists. When in training, one should start with easy cases such as small, unruptured ectopic pregnancies.

– The contraindications should be respected. The decision as to whether the approach should be conservative or radical will depend on the history of the patient and on her desire for further fertility.

TABLE 12.3 **Prognostic value of serial hCG determination after endosurgical treatment of ectopic pregnancy**

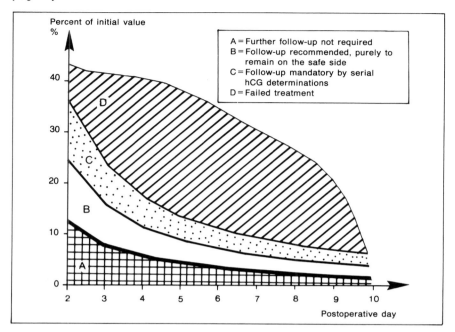

Fertility results

Fertility after treatment of ectopic pregnancy is a very real problem, especially in the developed countries, where an increase in the incidence of ectopic pregnancy is noted [25].

Among the 467 patients of this series (503 ectopic pregnancies), 223 had desire for further fertility and have been followed for more than a year. The others either used contraception (n = 167) or were lost to follow-up (n = 75).

Table 12.4 gives an overview of the results: 149 (67 %) had an intrauterine pregnancy, 6 of them following a recurrent ectopic that was also treated laparoscopically; 74 patients were considered sterile (32 %), 21 of them after a repeat ectopic pregnancy; 27 patients presented with a repeat extrauterine pregnancy (12 %).

TABLE 12.4 **Comparison between patients with differing histories with relation to postectopic fertility (for each patient only the first EP is considered)**

	Cases	IUP		EP		Infertility	
	N	N	%	N	%	N	%
Control group (group D)	101	91	90.0	5	5.0	5	5.0
EP group	31	8[a]	25.8	9[a]	29.0	14[a]	45.2
Solitary tube group	36	14[a]	38.9	11[b]	30.5	11[a]	30.5
Previous infertility	102	38[a]	37.2	18[b]	17.7	46[b]	45.1
Tubal infertility	62	16[a]	25.8	11[b]	17.8	35[a]	56.4
Nontubal infertility	40	22[a]	55.0	7[b]	17.5	11[a]	27.5
Salpingitis	29	11[a]	38.0	7[c]	24.0	11[b]	38.0

[a] $p < 0.001$.
[b] $p < 0.01$.
[c] $p < 0.05$.
Note: All statistical comparisons are made versus group D results.

The patient's history greatly influences the outcome. Four major groups have been distinguished: group A is composed of 101 patients with no previous history (infertility, ectopic pregnancy, salpingitis, or solitary tube); group B is made up of 122 patients with antecedents of infertility, ectopic pregnancy, salpingitis, or solitary tube.

In group A, intrauterine pregnancy occurred in 90 % of cases, with recurrence of ectopic pregnancy in 5 %. The figures in group B are, respectively, 42.6 % (p < 0.01) and 18 % (p < 0.01).

Our overall success rate is higher than most data reported in the literature (Tables 12.5 and 12.6). Comparison between the different series shows not only the large variability in results but also that endosurgical conservative treatment gives results compared to those obtained by techniques requiring laparotomy. This is particularly true for patients without a prior history of infertility, among whom a 90 % success rate is seen.

TABLE 12.5   **Literature overview of fertility outcome after treatment of ectopic pregnancy**

Author	Date	Number of patients	IUP N	IUP %	EUP N	EUP %
Conservative treatment						
Ploman [22]	1960	31	16	52	1	3.2
Skulj [28]	1964	92	23	25	1	1.1
Timonen [31]	1967	185	46	24.8	21	11.5
Palmer [21]	1972	55	11	20	9	17.5
Swollin [30]	1972	40	10	25	7	17.3
Jarvinen [14]	1972	43	22	51.2	4	9.3
Stromme [29]	1973	37	20	54.1	7	18.9
Bukowsky [2]	1979	20	14	70	1	5
De Cherney [6]	1979	48	19	39	4	8
Giana [9]	1979	51	17	33	4	7.8
Henri-Suchet [12]	1979	52	22	42	10	19
Sherman [27]	1982	47	39	83	7	15.5
Lalau [16]	1985	118	35	29.6	29	24.7
Microsurgery						
De Cherney [7]	1980	9	5	55	0	0
Janecek [13]	1980	10	6	60	2	20
Endosurgery						
Author's data	1989	223	149	67	27	12

The good results are explained by

– Earlier diagnosis, due to use of hCG and ultrasonography, which has allowed better results independent of the technique used [11, 18, 28].

– Improvements we have brought to conservative surgical treatment performed at laparotomy or laparoscopy:

- Chemical hemostasis with vasopressin, eliminating traumatic methods of stopping bleeding, such as coagulation or suturing.
- Elimination of suturing of the incision in the tubal wall, lowering the risk of secondary occlusion. The studies of Gordji [10] and McComb [17] have shown that omission of suturing allows more physiologic repair, especially concerning orientation of mucosal folds. In two-thirds of cases, healing reconstitutes all three layers of the tube. In one-third of cases, only the mucosa and serosa close, causing a "tubal hernia," which does not seem to influence tubal physiology. We detected one case of fistula in a patient treated twice at the same site.

– Advantages of laparoscopy:

- Manipulation is kept to a minimum; trauma to the affected tube is minimal and to the contralateral tube nonexistent.
- Adhesion formation is less prevalent after laparoscopic surgery. In our first 18 patients, we performed a second-look laparoscopy and could find adhesions in only 5 cases. Adhesions are notoriously the cause of infertility following treatment of ectopic pregnancy. The aim of the treatment should be to limit adhesion formation to a minimum. Adhesions can, of course, preexist surgery or be caused by it. Ryan [24] showed that the presence of fresh blood does not cause adhesions unless associated with dryness of the peritoneum, a condition that is virtually nonexistent in laparoscopy. Microsurgical techniques also tend to lower the drying of tissues. Laparoscopy, in addition, eliminates airborne contamination and other factors—such as gauze, towels, and talc from surgical gloves—leading to adhesions.

TABLE 12.6 **Literature overview of fertility outcome after treatment of ectopic pregnancy in patients with "single tube"**

Author	Date	Number of patients	IUP		EUP	
			N	%	N	%
Ploman [22]	1960	7	3	43	2	28
Mintz [20]	1962	25	8	32	3	12
Jarvinen [14]	1972	10	6	60	3	30
Stromme [29]	1973	5	2	40	2	40
Bukowsky [2]	1979	2	1	100	0	0
Giana [9]	1979	2	1	50	0	0
Henri-Suchet [12]	1979	14	8	57	2	15
De Cherney [5]	1982	15	8	53	3	20
Author's data		36	14	38.9	11	30.5

12.16–12.18 When the hematosalpinx is chronic, the Triton is not useful. The pregnancy must then be removed with the help of graspers.

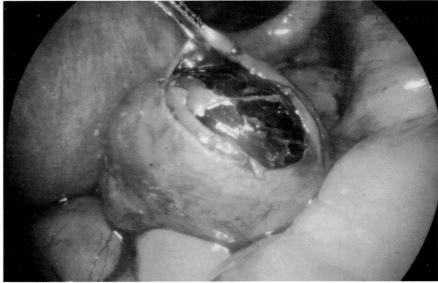

12.16

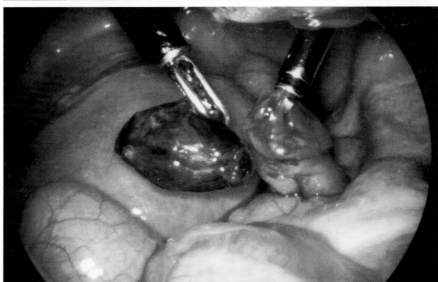

12.17

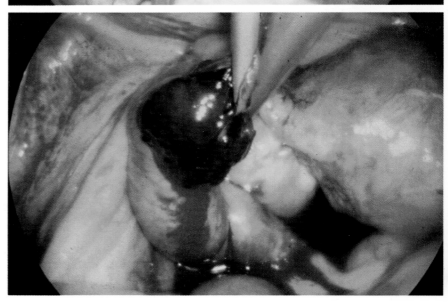

12.18

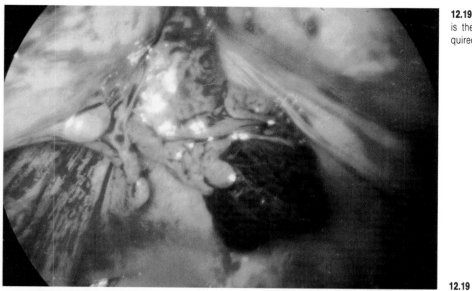

12.19 and 12.20 Fimbrial ectopic pregnancy. This is the only case in which salpingotomy is not required.

12.19

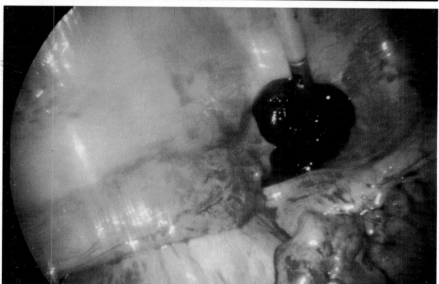

12.20

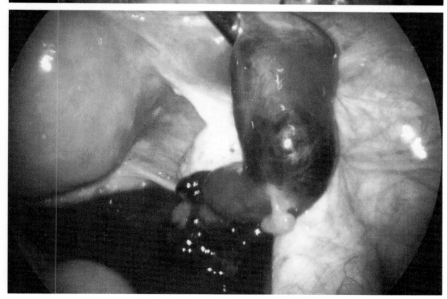

12.21 Ectopic pregnancy with perfusion disorder of the fallopian tube. The use of ornipressin is not indicated in this case.

Indications and contraindications for conservative treatment (Figs. 12.27 through 12.30)

Contraindications

Absolute contraindications

- Hemorrhagic shock
- Hemoperitoneum of more than 2000 mL
- Uncontrollable hemorrhage
- Hematocele
- Interstitial ectopic pregnancy
- Conditions unfavorable for laparoscopy (extensive adhesions)

Contraindications for conservative surgery

- Tubal pregnancy of 6 cm diameter or larger
- hCG titers above 20,000 IU/mL
- Patients at a high risk for recurrence

Indications

Since 1983, the proportion of ectopic pregnancies treated by laparoscopy in our department has exceeded 90 %. This figure represents a maximum, because we have a team very well trained in laparoscopic surgery. Seventy-five to 80 % is probably a more realistic figure.

The laparoscopic approach to treatment of ectopic pregnancy has several advantages over classical treatment by laparotomy. The operating time is shorter, the inherent complications of laparotomy are avoided, fertility is preserved as well if not better than after treatment by laparotomy and, finally, the hospital stay is significantly reduced. This represents a reduction in cost, largely balancing the cost of the equipment needed. The following criteria have been formulated.

- Failure rate: The failure rate is probably less than 2 % if the indications are respected. Failure can be anticipated as early as the second postoperative day and adequate treatment initiated. This is done by laparotomy, repeat laparoscopy, or perhaps with drugs such as methotrexate or RU 486. The failure rate of conservative treatment by laparotomy is estimated to be 1 % [15].

- Recurrence rate: The incidence of recurrence is quite high in our series. However, our data reflect the inclusion of a good many cases from the early years, for whom we would now advise in vitro fertilization (IVF). Recently, our recurrence rate has dropped to 10 %, with an unchanged success rate.

Conservative surgical treatment is a good approach for most of the following:

- Patients without a prior history of infertility
- Patients wearing an IUCD or desiring sterilization, because tubal ligation can be performed concomitantly
- Patients who have previously undergone several surgical procedures for reconstruction, as a tubal ligation can be done and, subsequently, IVF.

Site of implantation

The site of implantation influences the technique applied only slightly. In our series, the incidence of intrauterine pregnancy was 60.4 %, 61.2 %, or 84.2 % when the ectopic pregnancy was located in the isthmus, ampulla, or fimbria, respectively. Only the fimbrial site leads to significantly different results, but all results are satisfactory. The recurrence rate is 18 %, 11.2 %, and 5.3 %, respectively. These rates are not statistically different ($0.1 > p > 0.5$).

An isthmic location often leads to rupture. Use of POR 8 allows hemostasis in all cases. Postoperative tubal obstruction is more frequent than for other implantation sites and may sometimes require anastomosis. However, if the contralateral tube is intact, a normal intrauterine pregnancy may occur. Alternatively, one can perform partial resection and reanastomosis, which is quite difficult.

The ampullary location is the most common. Treatment by laparoscopic surgery is then limited by the size of the hematosalpinx and the extent of the hemoperitoneum.

The fimbrial location does not present any difficulty for conservative surgery, and results are particularly good. Ovarian pregnancy (Figs. 12.22, 12.23, 12.24) can also be treated by laparoscopy. POR 8 is injected along the ovarian and infundibulopelvic ligaments; then the pregnancy and blood clots are removed by aspiration.

Rupture

Rupture of the pregnant tube does not bear any consequences in terms of recurrence or success rates. The intrauterine pregnancy rate in case of rupture is 62.9 % versus 64.6 % in the absence of rupture; the recurrence rates are 14.5 % and 11.2 %, respectively. We had anticipated a higher difference. The absence of difference is probably due to the advantages of laparoscopy; namely, fewer postoperative adhesions and less trauma to the unaffected tube [17].

Ectopic pregnancy score

Indications for conservative treatment depend more on the history of the patient than on the type of ectopic pregnancy. We developed a score based on a multifactorial analysis of our results, taking into account which parameters significantly affected the fertility results. The statistical weight of the risk factors and the therapeutic score of EP are as follows:

Score data	Score	Statistical weight
One previous ectopic pregnancy	2	0.434
For each additional ectopic pregnancy[a]	1	0.261
Previous laparoscopic adhesiolysis[b]	1	0.258
Previous tubal microsurgery[b]	2	0.351
Solitary tube	2	0.472
Previous salpingitis	1	0.242
Homolateral adhesions	1	0.207
Contralateral adhesions[c]	1	0.198

[a] If the ectopic occurred in both tubes, just count "solitary tube."
[b] Only one is taken in count.
[c] If the tube is blocked or absent, count "solitary tube."

Each patient then was scored by adding up the weight of each risk factor. We then confronted this score with all our cases, studying the rates of IUP, recurrence, and infertility. Table 12.7 clearly shows that the IUP rate decreases inversely with the score, whereas the rates for recurrence and infertility increase. There comes a point, at a score of 4, where the risk of EP is equivalent to that of IUP. For higher scores, the risk of recurrence is dramatically higher than the probability of an IUP. Therefore, based on this analysis, the following treatment recommendations are made according to the total risk score:

- Score 0 to 4: conservative laparoscopic treatment
- Score 5: radical laparoscopic treatment consisting of salpingectomy
- Score 6 and above: radical laparoscopic treatment with contralateral sterilization and recommendation to enter an IVF program

TABLE 12.7 **Probability of IUP and risk of EP according to the score (expected and observed data)**

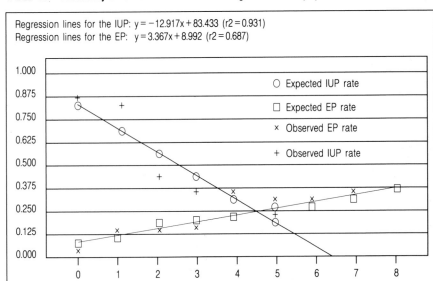

Regression lines for the IUP: $y = -12.917x + 83.433$ ($r2 = 0.931$)
Regression lines for the EP: $y = 3.367x + 8.992$ ($r2 = 0.687$)

○ Expected IUP rate
□ Expected EP rate
× Observed EP rate
+ Observed IUP rate

Second-look laparoscopy (Figs. 12.31 through 12.33)

In view of the rather good results of conservative treatment for ectopic pregnancy, second-look laparoscopy is indicated only in selected cases. Hysterosalpingography brings little informaltion for evaluation of the risk of recurrence, and laparoscopy is too invasive to be performed systematically. We advise second look only in the following cases:

- One year or more of infertility posttreatment
- Presence of adhesions at the time of treatment
- Need for reconstructive surgery of the contralateral tube

Conclusion

Conservative treatment at laparoscopy for ectopic pregnancy has proved to be safe and successful in terms of eliminating the products of conception and preserving fertility. It is possible in approximately 80 % of cases of ectopic pregnancy. It requires respect for technique and contraindications, use of adequate instrumentation and, above all, expertise in laparoscopic surgical procedures.

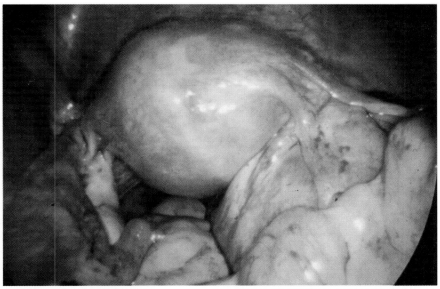

12.22 and 12.23 Large ovarian pregnancy, which is treated by aspiration.

12.22

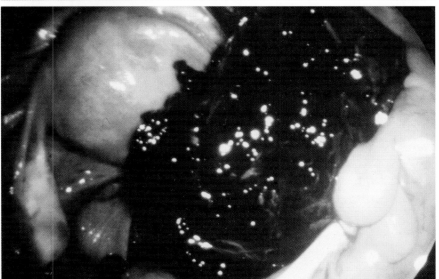

12.23

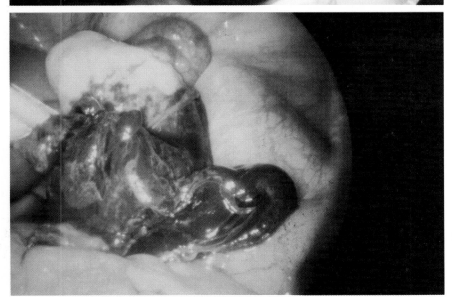

12.24 Another example of ovarian pregnancy.

12.25 and 12.26 Tubal pregnancy implanted at the ampullary isthmic junction. The lesion is quite small and could easily be missed if no systematic exploration is performed.

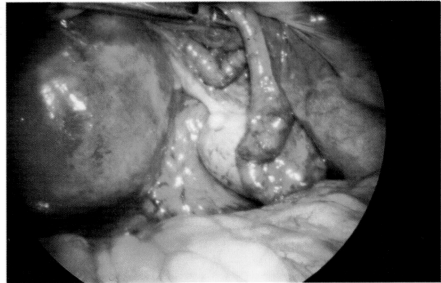

12.25

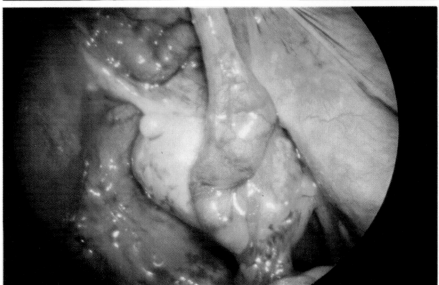

12.26

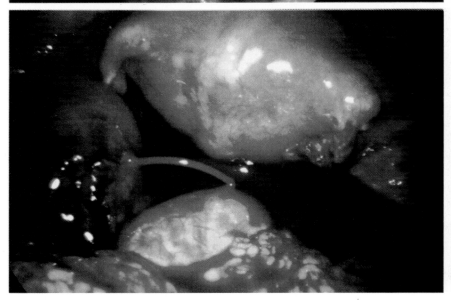

12.27 Arterial bleeding from an ectopic pregnancy. Endosurgical treatment is abandoned if the bleeding cannot be controlled quickly.

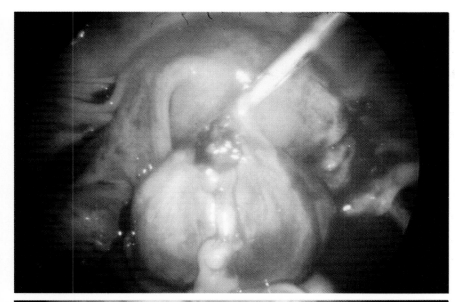

12.28 Large ruptured ectopic pregnancy. An embryo can be seen hanging on its umbilical cord (lower border of the illustration). Laparoscopic treatment is contraindicated.

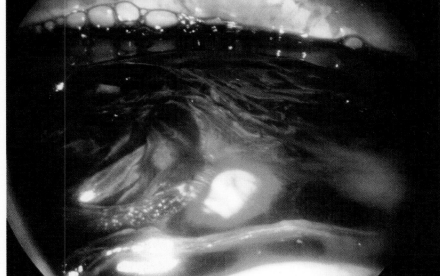

12.29 A massive hemoperitoneum represents a contraindication to endosurgical treatment.

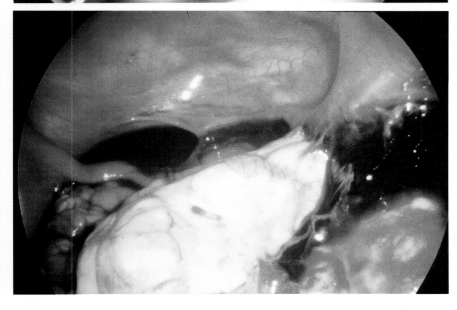

12.30 A hematocele is also a contraindication for laparoscopic surgery.

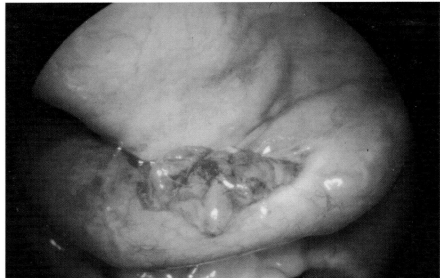

12.31 Protrusion of the mucosal folds through the incision after extraction of the products of conception. These folds need to be excised or repositioned within the lumen.

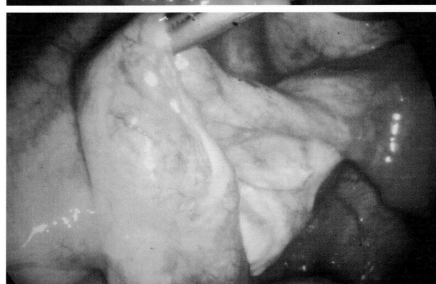

12.32 Typical appearance of the tubal scar after endosurgical treatment of an ectopic pregnancy.

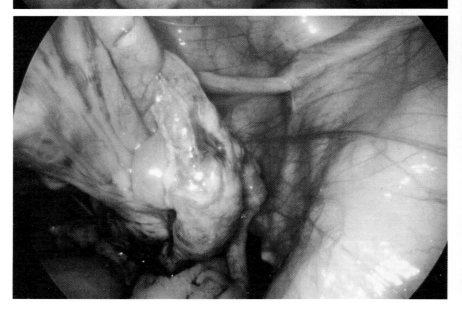

12.33 Adhesion formation involving the incision site after laparoscopic treatment of an ectopic pregnancy.

References

1. Bruhat M.A., Manhes H., Mage G., Pouly J.L., « Treatment of ectopic pregnancy by means of laparoscopy », *Fertil. Steril.*, 1980; 33 : 411.
2. Bukowsky I., Langer R., Sherman A., Caspi E., « Conservative surgery for ectopic pregnancy », *Obstet. Gynecol.*, 1979; 53 : 709.
3. Curran P.W., « Economic consequence of pelvic inflammatory disease in the United States », *Am. J. Obstet. Gynecol.*, 1980; 138 : 848.
4. Collège national des gynécologues et obstétriciens français. Résultats bruts de l'enquête: « Evaluation de la fréquence des GEU en France », *J. Gynecol. Obstet. Biol. Reprod.*, 1983; 12 : 325.
5. De Cherney A.H., Maheaux R., Naftolin F., « Salpingotomy for ectopic pregnancy in the sole patent oviduct: reproductive outcome », *Fertil. Steril.*, 1982; 37 : 619.
6. De Cherney A.H., Kase N., « The conservative surgical management of unruptured ectopic pregnancy », *Obstet. Gynecol.*, 1979; 54 : 451.
7. De Cherney A.H., Polan M.L., Kort H., Kase N., « Microsurgical technique in the management of tubal ectopic pregnancy », *Fertil. Steril.*, 1980; 34 : 324.
8. Dubuisson J.B., Aubriot F.X., Cardone V., « Laparoscopic salpingectomy for tubal pregnancy », *Fertil. Steril.*, 1987; 47 : 225.
9. Giana M., « Tratamento chirurgico conservativo in 51 caza du gravidenza tubarica », *Minerva Gynecol.*, 1979; 30 : 99.
10. Gordji M., Henri-Suchet J., Pigeaud F. et al., « Etude comparée des salpingotomies avec et sans suture. Recherche microchirugicale expérimentale sur la trompe de lapine », *J. Gynecol. Obstet. Biol. Reprod.*, 1981; 10 : 765.
11. Grant A., « The effect of ectopic pregnancy on fertility », *Clin. Obstet. Gynaecol.*, 1962; 5 : 861.
12. Henri-Suchet J., « Chirurgie conservatrice de la grossesse extra-utérine », In « Oviducte et fertilité », Masson, Paris, 1979, p. 393.
13. Janecek J., « Résultats de la chirurgie reconstructice dans les grossesses extra-utérines non rompues », *Rev. Med. Suisse Romande*, 1979; 99 : 603.
14. Jarvinen P.A., « Conservative operative treatment of tubal pregnancy with post-operative daily hydrotubation », *Acta Obstet. Gynecol. Scand.*, 1972; 51 : 169.
15. Kelly R.W., Martin S.A., Strickler R.C., « Delayed hemorrhage in conservative surgery for ectopic pregnancy », *Am. J. Obstet. Gynecol.*, 1979; 133 : 225.
16. Lalau Keraly M. (Madelenat P.), « Récidives de grossesse extra-utérine. A propos d'une étude multicentrique de 470 cas de GEU », Thèse, Paris, 1985.
17. McComb P., Gomel V., « Linear ampullary salpingotomy heals better by secondary versus primary closure », *Fertil. Steril.*, 1984; 41 : 45.
18. Mage G., Manhes H., Pouly J.L., Ropert J.F., Bruhat M.A., « Etude de la fertilité après traitement cœlioscopique de la grossesse tubaire non rompue », *J. Gynecol. Obstet. Biol. Reprod.*, 1983; 12 : 775.
19. Manhes H., Mage G., Pouly J.L., Ropert J.F., Bruhat M.A., « Traitement cœlioscopique de la grossesse extra-utérine non rompue: améliorations techniques », *Nouv. Presse Med.*, 1983; 12 : 1431.
20. Mintz M., « La chirurgie de la trompe gravide: 17 interventions et revue de la littérature », *Obstet. Gynecol.*, 1962; 61 : 385.
21. Palmer R., « Résultats et indications de la chirurgie conservatrice au cours de la grossesse extra-utérine », *C.R. Soc. Fr. Gynecol.*, 1972; 42 : 317.
22. Ploman L., Wicksell F., « Fertility after conservative surgery in tubal pregnancy », *Acta Obstet. Gynecol. Scand.*, 1960; 39 : 143.
23. Pouly J.L., Gachon M., Gaillard G., Mage G., Bruhat M.A., « La décroissance de l'HCG après traitement cœlioscopique conservateur de grossesse extra-utérine », *J. Gynecol. Obstet. Biol. Reprod.*, 1987; 16 : 195.
24. Ryan G.B., Grobety J., Majno G., « Postoperative peritoneal adhesions », *Am. J. Pathol.*, 1971; 65 : 117.
25. Schencker J.G., Evron S., « New concepts in the surgical management of ectopic pregnancy and the consequent postoperative results », *Fertil. Steril.*, 1983; 40 : 709.
26. Semm K., Mettler L., « Technical progress in pelvic surgery via operative laparoscopy », *Am. J. Obstet. Gynecol.*, 1980; 138 : 121.
27. Sherman D., Langer R., Sadovsky G., Bukovsky I., Capsi E., « Improved fertility following ectopic pregnancy », *Fertil. Steril.*, 1982; 37 : 497.
28. Skulj V., « Conservative operative treatment of tubal pregnancy », *Fertil. Steril.*, 1964; 15 : 634.
29. Stromme W.B., « Conservative surgery for ectopic pregnancy », *Obstet. Gynecol.*, 1973; 41 : 251.
30. Swollin K., Fall M., « Ectopic pregnancy », *Acta Eur. Fertil.*, 1972; 3 : 147.
31. Timonen S., Nieminen U., « Tubal pregnancy, choice of operative method of treatment », *Acta Obstet. Gynecol. Scand.*, 1967; 46 : 327.
32. Weström L., « Effect of acute pelvic inflammatory disease on fertility », *Am. J. Obstet. Gynecol.*, 1975; 121 : 707.

13

Assisted reproductive technology

Assisted reproductive technology has profoundly changed management of infertility during the last decade. Laparoscopy has played an important role [29]. This chapter will deal mainly with the operative techniques, ignoring the biological aspects, which are beyond the scope of this manual. The chapter is divided into three parts:
- Follicle puncture
- Intratubal transfer
- Other techniques

Follicle puncture

Laparoscopy was the first method employed to access the ovaries for follicle puncture [30] and, despite the advent of ultrasonography, it retains an important place.

Procedure

Mobilization of the ovary (Figs. 13.1, 13.2, and 13.3)

For access to the entire surface of the ovary, it is necessary to stabilize it with a flat forceps applied to the ovarian ligament. Access is gained through a midline trocar to reach both ovaries easily. The ovary can be maintained in a position such that the needle can approach at the appropriate angle. The forceps also permits rotation upward and laterally for access to the lateral side of the ovary.

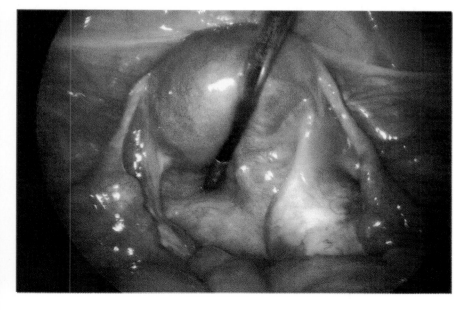

13.1 Laparoscopy for follicle puncture.

13.2 and 13.3 Rotation of the ovary for optimal access to all follicles is made possible by applying a forceps on the ovarian ligament.

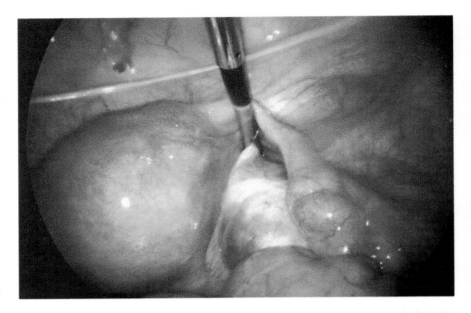

13.2

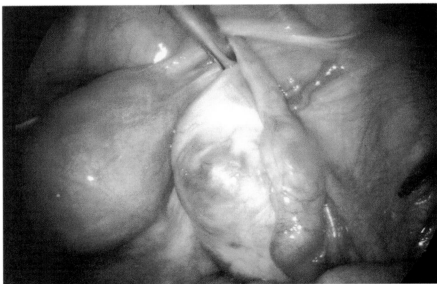

13.3

The puncture needle

Reseach by the pioneers in follicle puncture has delineated the important characteristics of the needle: the inner diameter must be 1 mm or more. Renou [28] and Jones [20] have shown identical results with needles of 1.0 and 2.2 mm in inner diameter. The bevel of the needle is 45° to 60°.

Method of aspiration

The negative pressure for optimal aspiration is between 80 and 120 mmHg, depending on the diameter of the needle. The needle is connected to a vial which, in turn, is connected to the aspiration system, equipped with a manometer. The connecting tubing is of a small diameter to reduce the dead space. Direct aspiration with a syringe does not allow control of the negative pressure, which, in the latter case, is higher than ideally permitted, leading to damage of the oocytes [7].

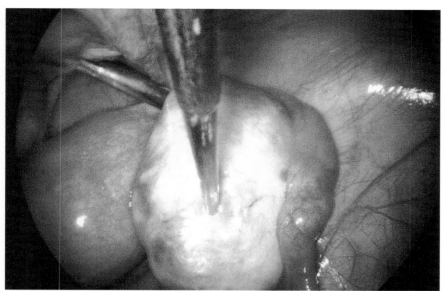

13.4

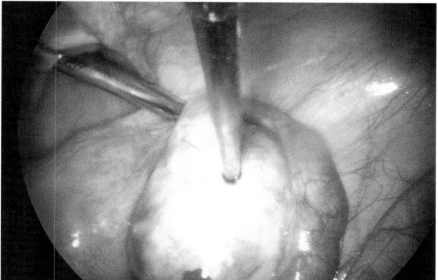

13.5

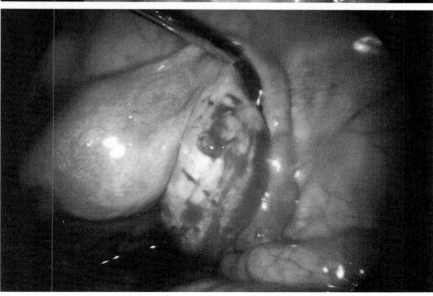

13.6 Appearance at completion of the procedure.

Holding the bowel back

Loops of bowel in the cul-de-sac often restrict access to the ovary. Bowel can be pushed out of the way either by transiently increasing the Trendelenburg position or by grasping one of the appendices epiploicae with an atraumatic forceps at the level of the rectosigmoid and pushing the rectosigmoid cephalad. Often the bowel will remain out of the way. Otherwise, the forceps is left in place and a supplementary trocar inserted. This scenario is particularly frequent in obese patients.

Difficult puncture

Most commonly, the ovary is difficult to approach because of multiple adhesions with omentum or bowel. When the ovary is fixed to the broad ligament, the follicles of the lateral side cannot be approached. In these cases, a compromise must be made between maximum pickup rate and the risk of injury by puncture through ill-defined structures. Adhesiolysis prior to puncture is sometimes unavoidable but often leads to premature rupture of the mature follicles.

Indications for laparoscopic puncture

Ultrasonographically guided puncture is currently the dominant method, but laparoscopy still has an important place for many teams. Laparoscopy is no longer used in our department because the pickup rate is greater with ultrasonography; moreover, fertilization is higher after ultrasonographically guided puncture, perhaps because of the absence of CO_2 from the pneumoperitoneum. However, the implantation rate is identical, independent of the method of follicle puncture.

The choice depends on three criteria.

Extent of adhesions

This is the prevalent criterion. Puncture of the follicles is then better performed under ultrasonographic control. This is also safer provided that only clearly identifiable structures are punctured. There have been reports of injury to the iliac vein, to the bowel, with subsequent peritonitis, and exitus. The technique of approach (transvaginal, urethral, or transvesical) should be chosen as to minimize risk to the patient [12, 16, 22, 26]. When the ovaries are not accessible ultrasonographically, laparoscopy is the method of choice for puncture of the follicles and for assessment of extent of adhesions.

Patient's preference

The patient's choice is influenced by past experience [4]. It is unfair to compare laparoscopy and general anesthesia with ultrasonography and local anesthesia [5]. Follicle puncture, either endoscopically or ultrasonographically, can be done with either local or general anesthesia. The choice, therefore, is composed of two decisions: (1) method of access and (2) method of analgesia. Patient motivation is the most important factor in the choice of anesthesia. Laparoscopy under local anesthesia is painful both pre- and postoperatively, compared to ultrasonographically guided puncture, which appears to us to be the best choice.

Associated procedures

Laparoscopy can have both diagnostic and therapeutic objectives, especially in the following situations:

— After tubal reconstructive surgery and a normal postoperative hysterosalpingogram when failure is thought to be due to adhesions, which could be resected during the laparoscopy [9].

— After surgical treatment of endometriosis where failure may be due to adhesion formation or to persistent disease, both of which can be treated surgically again at the time of laparoscopy [25].

Some procedures are possible, but absence of uterine manipulation impedes the surgery. The operator concedes more importance to the follicle puncture or to the operative procedure, in which case it is advisable to be able to freeze the embryos for transfer during a later cycle.

Adhesiolysis is performed after follicle puncture for two reasons:

— To facilitate further ovarian function. It is well demonstrated that encapsulated ovaries produce fewer follicles than do normal ovaries [23].

— To permit better access to the ovaries during a subsequent cycle.

Extremely extensive adhesions are, however, an indication for ultrasonographically guided puncture, which then means that it is not desirable to free the ovary from the broad ligament. In fact, these adhesions make puncture easier because the ovary is fixed in place.

In vitro fertilization at the time of diagnostic laparoscopy

Laparoscopy is required for every workup of infertility, and it may be tempting to take that opportunity for performing in vitro fertilization (IVF).

Combining diagnostic evaluation and IVF is done by some operators to limit the number of invasive procedures. Procedures such as adhesiolysis, salpingostomy, or resection of endometriotic implants can be done at the time of follicle puncture, but it is inconvenient [9, 10]. Intrauterine manipulation, required as adjuvant to surgical procedures, precludes embryo transfer during that same cycle. Embryos should be kept frozen for later transfer. Hyperstimulation of the ovaries makes adhesiolysis or treatment of ovarian endometriosis difficult. Moreover, this combination is not cost-effective, because the number of IVF cycles—which are quite expensive—is significantly increased. A well-performed laparoscopic surgery offers a chance of success equal to three or four IVF cycles. Moreover, once a patient is in an IVF program, it is difficult to convince her to terminate treatment [17].

The combination of diagnostic workup and IVF should, in our view, be done only in the following selected cases:

— Patients with previous tubal surgery or treatment of endometriosis with follow-up of at least 12 months. A laparoscopy, adhesiolysis or fimbrioplasty can be performed. This avoids an additional operation in patients who have already had quite a number and in whom the indication for IVF is legitimate.

— Patients with unexplained infertility, when previous laparoscopy was performed several years before [3]. The laparoscopy is aimed at detecting pathology that has become apparent in the meantime.

Intratubal transfer

Gamete intrafallopian transfer (GIFT) was introduced by Asch [2, 3]. This procedure allows fertilization of oocytes by spermatozoa in a natural milieu and also permits migration to the uterine cavity in a physiologic way. Initial results are encouraging.

Procedure (Figs. 13.7, 13.8, and 13.9)

Follicle puncture is performed as previously described, via laparoscopy. Oocytes are then transferred to the tube in a catheter and mixed with 30 to 100×10^3 capacitated spermatozoa. The catheters must have 0.5 mm or more in internal diameter to be able to aspirate the oocyte with surrounding cumulus.

We use catheters intended for endotracheal aspiration in neonates; these are extremely supple and atraumatic. The catheter is introduced into the abdomen through a Thuohy needle (14 charrière). This gives the catheter a 30° angle when it exits the needle. The ampulla is held straight upward and the Thuohy needle inserted percutaneously approximately 1 cm above the projection of the ampulla. The catheter is pushed through the Thuohy needle 3 cm into the tubal lumen. The injected volume is approximately 40 to 120 μL, depending on the concentration of spermatozoa. The ampulla is held in the upright position for 2 min to allow elimination of bubbles and attachment of the cumulus to the tubal mucosa. Many commercial sets are available for GIFT.

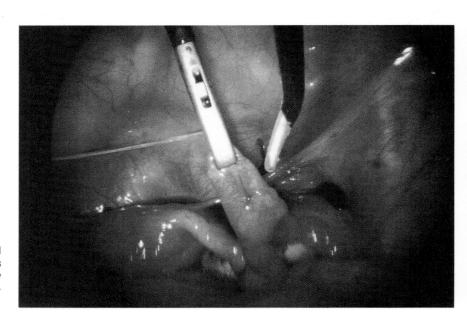

13.7 GIFT: The fimbriated end is grasped and held upward with graspers. The GIFT catheter is pointed toward the fimbriated end. The Thuohy needle has a beveled opening and therefore facilitates guidance of the catheter.

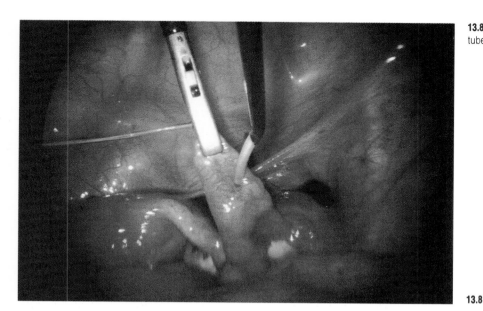

13.8 and 13.9 The catheter is advanced into the tube over a distance of approximately 3 cm.

13.8

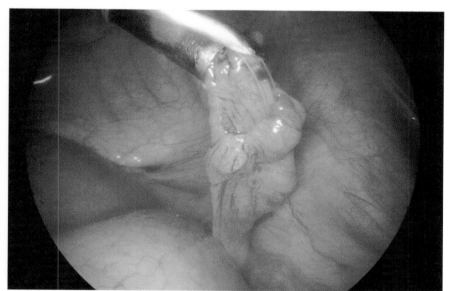

13.9

Indications

As for all new techniques, the indications of GIFT are not yet well defined. GIFT can be performed any time there is no increased risk for ectopic pregnancy. The method has the advantage that only a small number of spermatozoa are required; a pregnancy has been achieved with only 10,000. This technique also short-circuits the peritoneal fluid, which has a detrimental role in fertilization. Moreover the results of GIFT seem to be better than those of IVF. The method is used in the following cases:

    — Infertility due to endometriosis without tubal pathology.

    — Infertility due to antibodies in the cervical mucus.

    — Unexplained infertility [26].

    — Infertility after cone biopsy (absence of mucus and/or severe cervical stenosis).

– Infertility due to male factor. This appears to be a good indication, but opinions vary [24]. Asch [2] believes it to be a good indication; Cittadini disagrees [18]. In our opinion, there is no difference between GIFT and IVF in this situation. That is, we believe IVF is better than either, because it provides more information important for diagnosis [27]. Leeton arrived at the same conclusion [21].

– Finally, infertility due to multiple factors.

Results

The data reported indicate a 20 % to 30 % success rate, which is significantly higher than that for IVF; however, the patient selection is different. Comparison of IVF versus GIFT remains an area of controversy. Comparative studies will soon elucidate the question of respective indications.

Still, GIFT remains a cumbersome technique requiring strict coordination between physician and biologist and a close spatial relationship between the operating room and the laboratory. The laparoscopy must be well-planned, just as for IVF, and lasts 30 to 60 min. The biologist must retrieve the eggs and then place them in the catheters with the spermatozoa. Therefore the operation takes longer than for IVF, and the postoperative course is more painful than after follicle puncture for IVF only.

In 1987, Anderson retrieved and replaced oocytes under ultrasonographic control [1]. Thus far, his results have not been duplicated by other researchers. The advantage is that the entire procedure can be done with minimal analgesia. The disadvantage is that, as no laparoscopy is performed, there is no opportunity for an updated evaluation of the pelvis.

Other techniques and diagnostic tests

Zygote intrafallopian transfer (ZIFT)

When GIFT is performed, one does not know whether fertilization has actually taken place. IVF can be considered a diagnostic test of fertilization, especially in male infertility. The principle of ZIFT is that transfer is performed only after fertilization, in the pronucleus or four-cell stage. Obviously, in this case follicle puncture is performed under ultrasonographic control to avoid two subsequent general anesthesias. The technique and the indications are the same for GIFT, but ZIFT is especially indicated in the presence of antibodies in serum in the female. According to Devroey and Yovich, ZIFT of two to three zygotes is equivalent to the intrauterine transfer of 5 embryos in IVF [6, 13, 32].

Diagnostic tests

Laparoscopy is a very important test for evaluation of infertility, but for a long time the search was only for adhesions or endometriotic implants. However, tubal surgery, adhesiolysis, or resection of endometriotic tissue is not synonymous with fertility, even when an excellent anatomic result is obtained. Other biological mechanisms are involved. Peritoneal fluid probably plays an important role in reproduction, and this fluid can be sampled during laparoscopy.

Cytology of peritoneal fluid for detection of spermatozoa

Peritoneal fluid should be sampled during the periovulatory phase, a few hours following intercourse. The search for spermatozoa requires treatment of the fluid with saponine, which destroys the red blood cells, followed by centrifugation. A positive test indicates that the spermatozoa are capable of reaching the site of fertilization. It is important to perform this test when there is an indication of sperm-mucus incompatibility, especially in the presence of additional male factor. Of course, this test does not tell us anything about the survival of sperm in the peritoneal fluid or about their fertilizing capability.

Sperm survival test in peritoneal fluid

Peritoneal fluid is sampled around the time of ovulation. After capacitation, the spermatozoa are incubated in the fluid at 37 °C in a 5 % CO_2 atmosphere. Mobility of the sperm is then measured at 1, 4, 8 and 24 h. Rapid decay of mobility is interpreted as an indication of a noxious substance in the peritoneal fluid, which would inhibit pickup of spermatozoa by the fimbriae and reduce chances of fertilization. The pathophysiologic mechanisms of this immobilization are certainly multiple: macrophages, lower peroxidase activity, immunoglobulins, etc. [14, 15, 19].

This test is of interest in the following cases:
- Incompatibility between sperm and female mucus
- Infertility due to antibodies in female mucus or serum
- Asthenospermia
- Mild or moderate endometriosis
- Unexplained infertility

In the absence of immobilization of sperm in this test, one could consider performing intraperitoneal fertilization. This technique consists of injecting 1 to 10×10^6 spermatozoa, after capacitation, into the cul-de-sac by culdocentesis.

Obviously laparoscopy is not absolutely necessary for performing these tests. Sampling of peritoneal fluid can also be done by culdocentesis. On the other hand, in performing laparoscopy for infertility, one should investigate more than tubal patency.

Conclusion

Laparoscopy lost its leading role in IVF with the advent of ultrasonography for follicle puncture. It has since returned to center stage with the introduction of GIFT; however, the indications for this technique in assisted reproductive technology remain ill defined.

References

1. Anderson J.G., Jansen R.P.S., « Ultrasound-guided catheterization of the fallopian tube for the non-operative transfer of gametes and embryos », VIe World Congress: in vitro fertilization and alternate assisted reproduction, Jerusalem, April 1989.
2. Asch D.H., Ellsworth L.H., Balmaceda J.P., Wong P.C., « Pregnancy after translaparoscopic gamete intrafallopian transfer », *Lancet*, 1984; n° 1034.

3. Asch R.H., Balmaceda J.P., Ellsworth L.H., Wong P.C., « Preliminary experiences with gamete intrafallopian transfer (GIFT) », *Fertil. Steril.*, 1986; 45 : 366-371.
4. Belaisch-Allart J., Hazout A., Glissant M., Frydman R., « Comparaison des différentes méthodes de recueil des ovocytes en fécondation in vitro », *Contracept. Fertil. Sexual.*, 1986; 14 : 703-708.
5. Belaisch-Allart J., Guillet-Rosso F., Baton C., Champagne C., Bodereau A.M., Frydman R., « Cœlioscopie sous anesthésie locale pour recueil d'ovocytes en vue de fécondation in vitro », *Nouv. Presse Med.*, 1983; 12 : 2053-2054.
6. Blackledge D., Matson G., Willcox D.L. et coll., « Pronuclear stage transfer and modified gamete intrafallopian transfer techniques for oligospermic cases », *Med. J. Aust.*, 1986; 145 : 173-174.
7. Cohen J., Avery S., Campbell S. et coll., « Follicular aspiration using a syringe system may damage the zona pellucida », *J. In Vitro Fertil. Emb. Transf.*, 1986; 3 : 224-226.
8. Cohen J., Fehilly C., Fishel S.B., Edwards R.G., « Male infertility successfully treated by in vitro fertilization », *Lancet*, 1984; n° 1239-1240.
9. Daniell J.F., Pittaway D.E., Maxson W.S., « The role of laparoscopic adhesiolysis in an in vitro fertilization program », *Fertil. Steril.*, 1983; 40 : 49-52.
10. Daniell J.F., Herbert C.M., « Laparoscopic salpingotomy utilizing the CO_2 laser », *Fertil. Steril.*, 1984; 41 : 558.
11. De Kretsen D.M., Yates C., Kovacs G.T., « The use of IVF in the management of male infertility », *Clin. Obstet. Gynaecol.*, 1985; 12 : 767-773.
12. Dellenbach P., Nisand I. et coll., « Transvaginal sonographically controlled ovarian follicle puncture for retrieval », *Lancet*, 1984; n° 1467.
13. Devroey P., Broeckman P., Smith P. et coll., « Pregnancy after translaparoscopic zygote intrafallopian transfer on a patient with sperm antibodies », *Lancet*, 1986; 1 : 1329.
14. Dorez F., Cavaille F., Sureau C., « Hypothèses relatives aux variations de mobilité des spermatozoïdes dans le liquide péritonéal », *J. Gynecol. Obstet. Biol. Reprod.*, 1985; 14 : 955-958.
15. Forler A., « Liquide péritonéal et fertilité—Insémination intra-péritonéale par culdocenthèse», Thèse de Médecine, Université René-Descartes, Paris, 1986.
16. Gleicher N., Friberg J. et coll., «Egg retrieval for in vitro fertilization sonographically controlled vaginal culdocentesis», *Lancet*, 1983; n° 508-509.
17. Greenfeld D., Haseltine F., « Candidate selection and psychological considerations of in vitro fertilization procedures », *Clin. Obstet. Gynaecol.*, 1986; 29 : 119-126.
18. Guastella G., Comparetto G., Cittadini E. et coll., « Gamete intrafallopian transfer (GIFT): a new technique for the treatment of unexplained infertility », *Acta Europ. Fertil.*, 1985; 16 : 311-314.
19. Halme J., Hall J.L., « Effect of pelvic fluid from endometriosis patients on human sperm penetration of zona-free hamster ova », *Fertil. Steril.*, 1982; 37 : 573.
20. Jones H.W., Acosta A.A., Garcia J., « A technique for the aspiration of oocytes from human ovarian follicles », *Fertil. Steril.*, 1982; 37 : 26.
21. Leeton J., Rogers C., Healy D., Yates C., « A controlled study between the use of gamete intrafallopian transfer (GIFT) and in vitro fertilization and embryo transfer in idiopathic and male infertility », *Fertil. Steril.*, 1988; 48 : 605-607.
22. Lenz S., Lauritzen J.G., « Ultrasonically guided percutaneous aspiration of human follicules under local anesthesia. A new method of collecting oocytes for in vitro fertilization », *Fertil Steril.*, 1982; 38 : 673-681.
23. Mahadevan M.M., Wiseman D., Leader A., Taylor P., « The effects of ovarian adhesive disease upon follicular development in cycles of controlled stimulation for in vitro fertilization », *Fertil. Steril.*, 1985; 44 : 489-493.
24. Matson P.L., Blackledge D.G., Richardson P.A., Turner S.R., Yovich J.M., Yovich J.L., « The role of gamete intrafallopian transfer (GIFT) in the treatment of oligospermic infertility », *Fertil. Steril.*, 1988; 48 : 608-612.
25. Nezhat C., Crowgey S.R., Garrison C.P., « Surgical treatment of endometriosis via laser laparoscopy », *Fertil. Steril.*, 1986; 45 : 778-783.
26. Parson J., Booker M., Akkermans J., Riddle A., Sharma V., Wilson V., Whitehead M., Campbell S., « Oocyte retrieval for in vitro fertilization by ultrasonically guided needle aspiration via the urethra », *Lancet*, 1985; n° 1076.
27. Pouly J.L., Vye P., Janny L., Canis M., Bassil S., Gioanni G., « Comparaison entre la FIVETE et le GIFT dans les hypofertilités masculines », Présenté au 3e Séminaire Niçois de Reproduction, 30 Avril 1988.
28. Renou P., Trounson A.O., Wood C., Leeton J.F., « The collection of human oocytes for in vitro fertilization. An instrument for maximising oocyte recovery rate », *Fertil. Steril.*, 1981, 35 : 409-412.
29. Steptoe P.C., Edwards R.G., « Birth after reimplantation of a human embryo », *Lancet*, 1978; 2 : 366.
30. Steptoe P.C., Edwards R.G., « Laparoscopic recovery of preovulatory human oocytes after priming ovaries with human gonadotropins », *Lancet*, 1970; 1 : 683-689.
31. Trounson A.O., Leeton J.F., Wood C., Weeb J., Wood J., « The investigation of idiopathic infertility by in vitro fertilization », *Fertil. Steril.*, 1980; 34 : 431-438.
32. Yovich J.L., Yovich J.M., Edirisinghe W.R, « The relative chance of pregnancy following tubal or uterine procedures », *Fertil. Steril.*, 1988; 49 : 858.

14
Tubal ligation

Laparoscopy is currently the method of choice for tubal sterilization. There is an abundance of techniques. Although the objective is irreversible interruption of the tube, it is advisable to use methods that cause minimal damage. Indeed, the success of reanastomosis is directly related to the quality and length of remaining tube and therefore to the method of sterilization used.

Procedure

General principles

Laparoscopy is performed according to the usual principles except that it has been shown that local anesthesia and the single-puncture approach are as effective as general anesthesia and double puncture.

Anesthesia

Local anesthesia is possible when the following are present:
 - Optimal conditions for laparoscopy: no prior laparotomy, no obesity, no known pelvic pathology
 - An experienced surgeon
 - An anesthesiologist present in the room and mandatory venous access
 - Sharp Verres needle
 - Strict adherence to protocol
 - Limited volume of pneumoperitoneum and limited angle of Trendelenburg

Equipment

Sterilization is quite a simple procedure which can be achieved with a single-puncture technique. The combination instrument endoscope/ring applicator is the type distributed by the World Health Organization in developing countries.

Use of the suprapubic trocar allows a better visualization of the pelvis and is therefore to be preferred. The site of insertion of the suprapubic trocar depends on the particular conditions in each patient, keeping in mind that the instrument will have to be advanced at a right angle to the tube and that the left tube is always the most difficult to reach. We usually introduce the trocar in the midline.

A uterine manipulator is useful in all cases. If one wants to avoid its use—for example, patients at high risk for developing an infection (immunosuppression, cardiac valve disease)—a suprapubic probe can be used to lift the uterus.

Techniques

Monopolar electrocoagulation

Monopolar electrocoagulation was the first of all endoscopic sterilization methods. As for all uses of monopolar current, there is a risk for accidents due to the spread of the electrical current (intestinal or ureteral injury). Moreover, the destruction is quite extensive, and if the mesotubarian vessels are burned, the entire ampulla could necrose. All in all, monopolar coagulation is an unsatisfactory and relatively dangerous technique [8] which, in spite of good results (failure rate 0.35/1000) [13] (Fig. 14.1), should be abandoned.

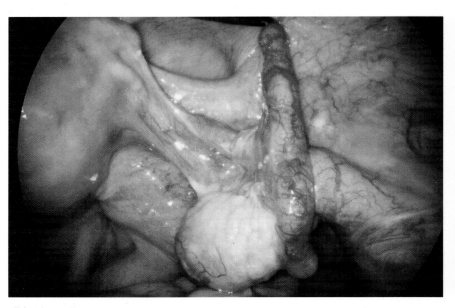

14.1 This figure illustrates the destruction caused by monopolar electrosurgery. The proximal portion of the oviduct as well as the mesosalpinx has disappeared. For this reason, in addition to the inherent potential hazards of electrosurgery, this method must be abandoned.

Bipolar electrocoagulation

Bipolar electrocoagulation only is insufficient. It must be followed by transection of the tube. Tissue damage is minimal if the mesotubarian vessels are not affected. Complications rarely occur. This method is rarely used in France but often in the United States (failure rate 1.1/1000) [4].

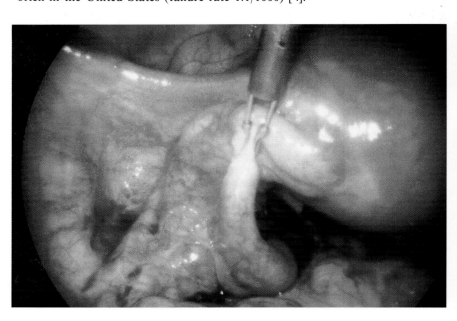

14.2 Bipolar desiccation of the oviduct leaves the vascularization intact.

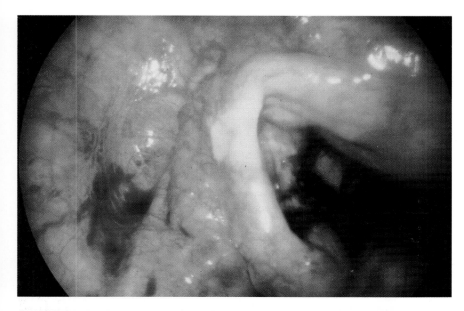

14.3 Appearance after desiccation.

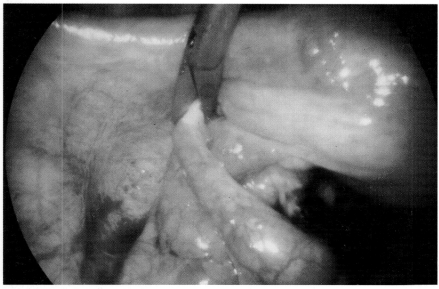

14.4 Cutting the tube in addition to desiccation is required for optimal results.

Thermocoagulation

This method was developed by Semm [7]. An application of 20 s at 120° to 140 °C is satisfactory (failure rate 0.21/1000) [9].

Yoon rings (Figs. 14.5 through 14.8)

This method, initially described by Yoon [11], rapidly became very popular. The rings have an external diameter of 3.5 mm and an internal diameter of 1.0 mm. They require a special applicator.

The ring is placed on the isthmus tubae, approximately 3 cm from the uterine horn, and a loop of tube, 1 to 1.5 cm, is pulled into the ring. The mesosalpinx is stretched by manipulating the uterus in the opposite direction, allowing approach of the tube at a right angle. The main complication is abruption of the tube, which can be avoided by a slow, progressive application. However, the fallopian tubes are sometimes thickened or edematous and must be ligated by another method. A ring can be applied on both stumps of the tube if rupture occurs. Incomplete occlusion is due to faulty application, which may explain a failure rate of 1 to 16/1000, depending on patient selection and the expertise of the operator [12].

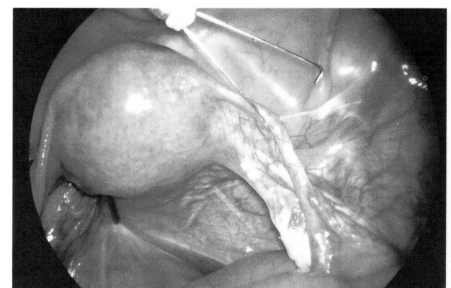

14.5 Prior to applying a ring, the tube is stretched to increase visualization of the mesosalpinx.

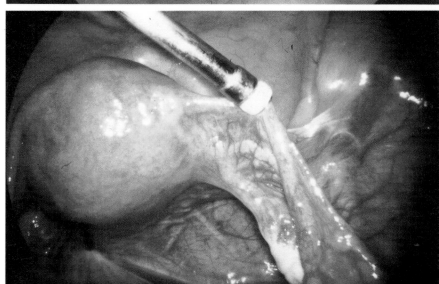

14.6 The tube is pulled into the probe slowly to avoid avulsion.

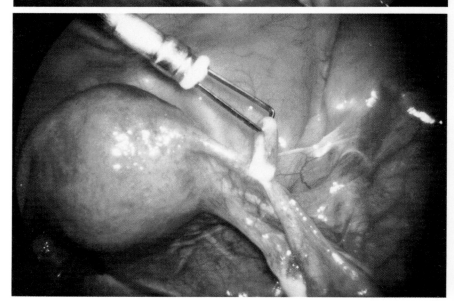

14.7 The first ring is put in place, closing onto a loop of approximately 1 cm of tube.

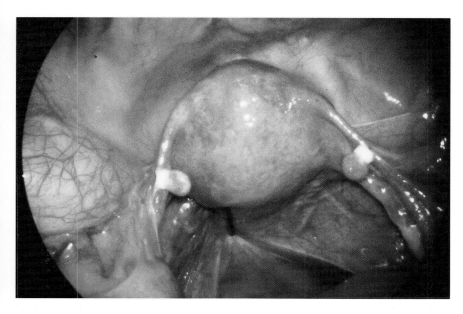

14.8 Final view: the rings are placed at approximately 2 cm from each uterine horn.

Clips (Figs. 14.9 through 14.12)

There are two different clips available: the Hulka-Clemens clip (1972) and the Filshie clip (1975). Tubal damage is least extensive with this method, and the application of the clips through suprapubic access is particularly easy. The operator must make sure that the clip encloses the entire diameter of the tube. Failure rate is less than 5 % for the Hulka clip [5] and between 0.9/1000 and 4.9/1000 for the Filshie clip [2] (not approved for use in the United States), which is the method we employ.

Filshie clip

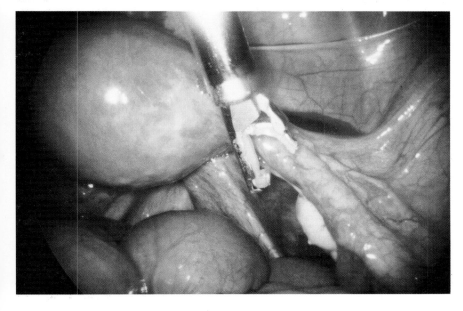

14.9 The mesosalpinx is stretched out, as for application of the Yoon ring. The long branch of the clip is placed along the posterior aspect of the mesosalpinx.

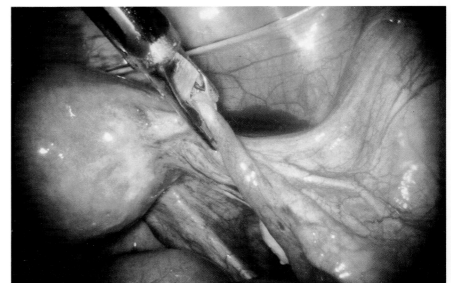

14.10 Closure of the clip transforms its shape, which is what keeps it on the tube and occludes the tube.

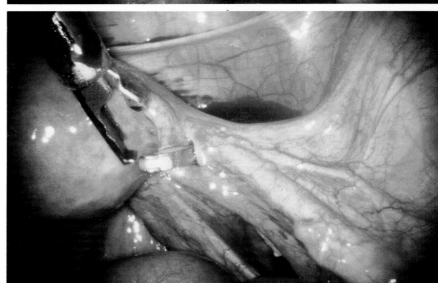

14.11 Situs after application of the first clip. Tubal damage is minimal; therefore we elected the Filshie clip as our method of choice.

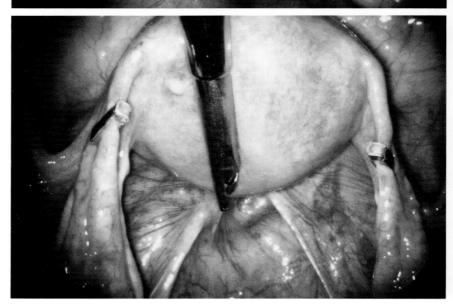

14.12 The applicator can be used as a probe for inspection of the pelvis.

Indications

There are two main indications for sterilization:
- Medical reasons
- Voluntary sterilization

The medical reasons correspond to absolute contraindications against carrying pregnancy to term. This is an important decision, made in concert with all specialists involved.

For voluntary sterilization, one should take the following into account:
- Age
- Parity
- Alternative contraception methods
- Psychological profile of the patient and her husband and estimation of the probability of regret [3].

Results

Overall, laparoscopic sterilization is a simple, safe, and effective operation. However, as for every surgical procedure, there is an incidence of morbidity and mortality and a failure rate.

Morbidity

Quite a number of national and international studies have shown that endoscopic tubal ligation is an effective method with a morbidity of 1 to 2 %, a figure clearly lower than that of laparotomy (5 to 10 %).

Risk factors are as follows:
- Patient-related: obesity, diabetes, prior pelvic surgery, or pelvic inflammatory disease (PID)
- Timing-related: postpartum, postabortion
- Operator-related: lack of experience in endoscopy
- Access-related: single-puncture approach has an incidence of morbidity approximately 16 times higher than the double-puncture approach
- Method-related: monopolar coagulation

Mortality

Mortality is not nil, but it is usually due to cardiovascular problems rather than to the procedure itself. The usual precautions must be observed. Monopolar coagulation should be abandoned in favor of mechanical methods such as the ring or clips.

Failure

The patient must be informed that intra- or extrauterine pregnancy can occur after sterilization. Failures can be divided into two categories:
- Method-related: faulty application of a ring or application onto the round ligament
- Luteal-phase pregnancy: the ligation was done in the luteal phase of the cycle

Monopolar coagulation has a higher incidence of fistulization [1]. When pregnancy occurs within the first year, it usually is intrauterine. The risk of ectopic pregnancy, as compared to intrauterine pregnancy, increases over time [10]. This risk of ectopic pregnancy also correlates with the existence of prior pelvic surgery or PID.

Recommendations to avoid failure

The following recommendations will likely lower the incidence of failure:
- Perform sterilization in the proliferative phase
- Use the second-puncture approach
- Identify the tubes accurately
- Apply the clip or ring correctly
- If the operator is a novice at laparoscopy, check the procedure carefully

Reversibility

An increase in the number of sterilizations has, of course, led to an increased demand for sterilization reversal. It is obvious that sterilization should be considered final, but it is equally obvious that the method used should allow conditions optimal for reversal. Extensive research has shown that reversal has the best chance for success when the segment of tube destroyed in the sterilization procedure was short. Currently it is estimated that clips destroy 5 to 7 mm; bipolar and endothermia, 15 to 20 mm; rings, 25 to 50 min; and, of course, monopolar, > 50 mm.

References

1. Cvigstad A., Jerve F., « Ectopic pregnancy following tubal sterilization », *Int. Fed. Gynecol. Obstet.*, 1982; 20 : 279-281.
2. Filshie G.M., « The Filshie clip », *In* « New Trends in Female Sterilization », Van Lith D.A.F., Keith L.G., Van Hall E.V.: Chicago, London: Year Book Medical, 1983; 115-124.
3. Hedon B., Denjean R., Damies J.P., Mares P., Valentin B., Viala J.L., Durand G., « Stérilités tubaires: Fécondation in vitro ou microchirurgie », *Presse Médicale*, 1989; 13 : 33-37.
4. Hirsch H.A., Nesser E., « Bipolar high frequency coagulation », *In* « New Trends in Female Sterilization », Van Lith D.A.F., Keith L.G., Van Hall E.V.; Chicago, London : Year Book Medical, 1983; 83-90.
5. Hulka J.F., Mercer J.P., Filshurne J.I. et al., « Spring clip sterilization: one-year follow-up of 1079 cases », *Am. J. Obstet. Gynecol.*, 1976; 125 : 1039.
6. Peterson H.B., Hulka F., Spelman F.J., Lee S., Marchbanks P.A., « Local versus general anesthesia for laparoscopic sterilization: a randomized study », *Obstet. Gynecol.*, 1987; 70 : 903.
7. Semm K., « Thermal coagulation for sterilization », *Endoscopy*, 1973; 5 : 218.
8. Soderström R.M., Yuzpe A.A., « Female sterilization », *Clin. Obstet. Gynaecol.*, 1979; 6 : 77-95.
9. Van Lith D.A.F., Van Schie K.J., Beetchuizen W., Binstock M., « Coagulation by the Semm and the Wolf techniques », *In* « New Trends in Female Sterilization », Van Lith D.A.F., Keith L.G., Van Hall E.V.; Chicago, London : Year Book Medical, 1983; 61-82.
10. Vessey M., Huggins G., Lawless M., Yeates D., « Tubal sterilization: findings in a large prospective study », *Br. J. Obstet. Gynaecol.*, 1983; 90 : 203-209.
11. Yoon I.B., King T.M., « A preliminary and intermediate report on a new laparoscopic tubal ring procedure », *J. Reprod. Med.*, 1975; 15 : 54.
12. Yoon I., Poliakoff S.R., « Laparoscopic tubal ligation: a follow-up report on the Yoon Falope ring procedure », *J. Reprod. Med.*, 1975; 15 : 54.
13. Yuzpe A.A., Rioux J.E., Loffer F.P., Pent D., « Laparoscopic tubal sterilization by the burn-only technique », *Obstet. Gynecol.*, 1977; 49 (1) : 106.

15

Uterine suspension

Laparoscopy for uterine suspension was described by Steptoe [9] and introduced in France by Abeille [1, 2]. This technique avoids laparotomy and is indicated primarily in the presence of chronic pelvic pain due to retroversion.

Endoscopic evaluation of retroversion (Figs. 15.1 and 15.2)

Diagnosis of chronic pelvic pain due to retroversion is essentially clinical; there is deep dyspareunia and the pain is reproducible at physical examination. There are also signs that can be detected at laparoscopy. First of all, there is the absence of any other pathology that could explain the chronic pelvic pain. Signs due to retroversion are dynamic, changing when the uterus is forced into anteversion. This dynamic change is an argument in favor of correcting the position of the uterus and permits the surgeon to evaluate the effect of the surgery.

Initially, the position of the uterus as seen through the laparoscope confirms the retroversion. The uterus has a typically mottled aspect and the infundibulopelvic ligaments present prominent venous vasodilation, the extent of

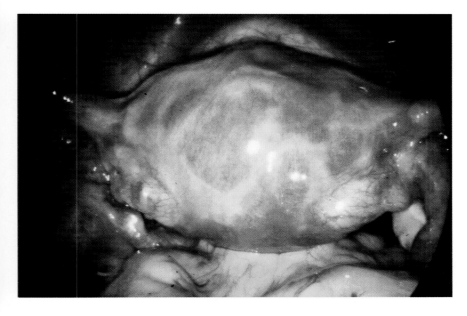

15.1 Retroverted uterus at the start of the procedure: note the mottled aspect, resulting from vascular dystrophy.

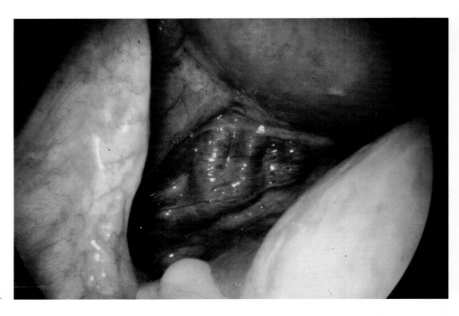

15.2 Large varicocele of the uterine pedicle.

which is often asymmetrical. Once the retroversion is corrected, inspection of the cul-de-sac will show:
   – Venous dilatation of one or both uterine pedicles
   – Modified appearance of the cul-de-sac, molded onto the retropositioned uterus

A few minutes after the uterus is positioned in anteversion, the corpus achieves a normal appearance and the venous dilatation recedes—good prognostic factors for the relief of chronic pain.

Procedure

The objective is to shorten the round ligaments in order to force the uterus into anteversion. Shortening should follow the anatomic course of the round ligament. Therefore it is important to know the anatomy of the inguinal canal.
   – The internal orifice of the inguinal canal is located about 1.5 cm above the inguinal ligament, midway between the anterior iliac spines and the pubis.
     – Important vessels are
        • Epigastric vessels, which run medially from the internal orifice and then cephalad in between the umbilical ligament and the lateral border of the rectus muscle
        • External iliac vessels, which describe a sharp angle with the epigastric vessels in a sagittal plane
   – The intra-abdominal course of the round ligament is oblique inward and dorsal, in a plane approximately perpendicular to the one made by the epigastric and iliac vessels.

Vascular injury is uncommon during this procedure, but it is important to have a good insight into the anatomy of the lower abdominal wall for maximum safety.

Incisions (Figs. 15.3 and 15.4)

Incision of the skin should theoretically be done at the level of the internal orifice of the inguinal canal. For cosmetic reasons, we make the incision more medial and lower, into the pubic-hair area. By blunt dissection, while the skin is retracted laterally, the fascia is reached. The two lateral incisions must be symmetrical. The genitofemoral nerve could be injured if the incision were made too high, with subsequent paresthesia.

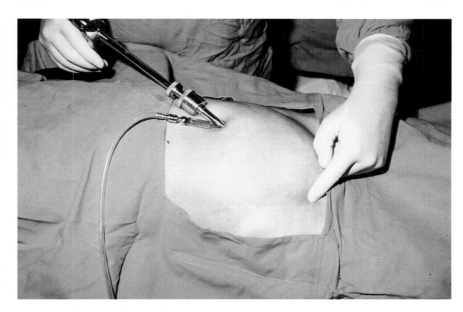

15.3 Locating the sites of incision.

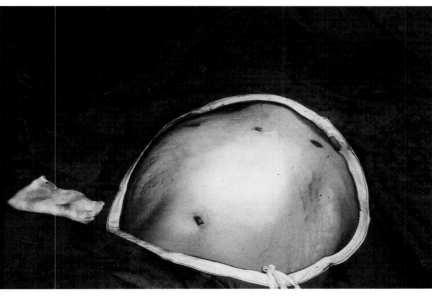

15.4 Incision sites at the end of the procedure.

Finding the internal inguinal ring (Figs. 15.5, 15.6, and 15.7)

A closed forceps, Bengolea or curved Kelly, is introduced with the tip of the forceps lateral to the epigastric vessels and facing the endoscope. Thereafter, the forceps is introduced further either retro- or intraperitoneally. This is of no importance, in our opinion. Indeed, the intraperitoneal technique does not lead to formation of peritoneal bridges that can possibly cause internal herniation.

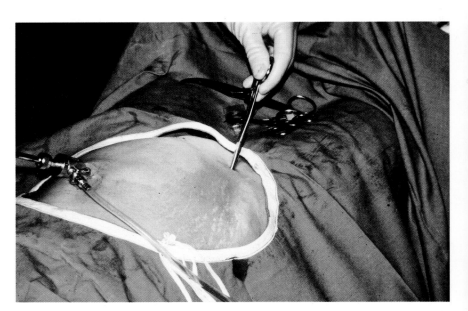

15.5 Insertion of a Kelly forceps through the suprapubic incision.

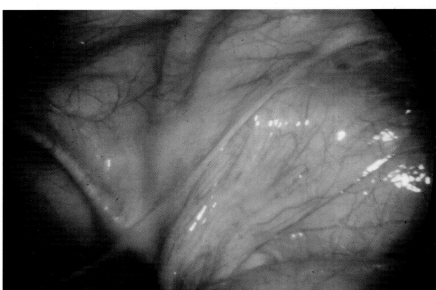

15.6 and 15.7 The forceps should enter the abdominal cavity through the inguinal ring, lateral to the ligament of Hasselbach.

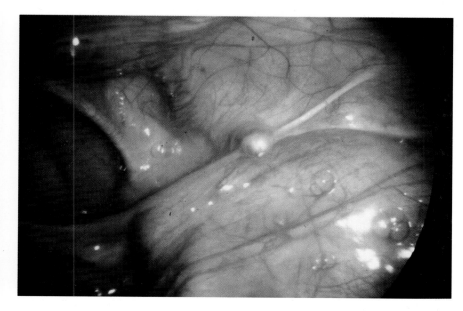

15.7

Grasping the round ligament (Figs. 15.8 through 15.11)

During insertion, the tip of the forceps is directed cephalad. Before grasping the round ligament, the forceps is turned so that the tip is now facing the hollow of the sacrum. This brings the forceps to a right angle with the round ligament, allowing a precise grasp without interfering with structures such as the mesosalpinx. The round ligament is grasped arbitrarily in the middle. If it appears that traction is excessive or asymmetrical, one can replace the forceps more laterally. The grip on the ligament should not be too tight, so as to avoid brittleness of the ligament in case the grip is placed more laterally. An inexperienced surgeon should place the two forceps before suturing, so that the suspension is symmetrical. Uterine manipulation helps to shorten the ligaments without placing excessive force on the sutures. The ligament rarely breaks. If it does, the proximal stump is grasped and sutured to the fascia. Optimal traction is that which is sufficient for the intra-abdominal pressure to keep the uterus in anteversion. Excessive traction should be avoided.

Suturing the round ligament (Figs. 15.11 and 15.12)

The ligament is sutured underneath the fascia of the rectus muscle with nonresorbable or slowly resorbable material. We usually apply two sutures in "X" or "U". The portion of the ligament that was pulled outside the peritoneal cavity should remain beneath the fascia to avoid painful herniation of the ligament. Also, sutures should be placed so that they do not cause necrosis of the ligament. Then the fascia is closed if necessary. The anatomic result is checked by laparoscopy at the end of the procedure. This is a simple procedure which requires no more than 10 min for an experienced surgeon.

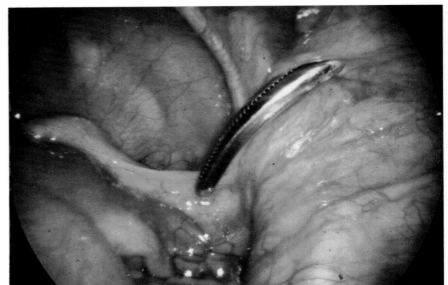

15.8 The round ligament is grasped medial to the iliac vessels.

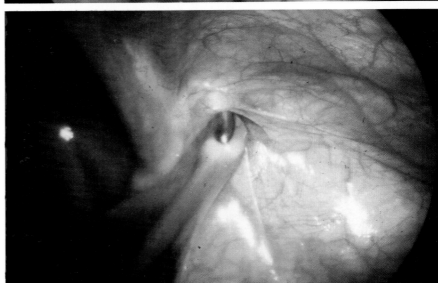

15.9 The round ligament is then pulled through the abdominal wall.

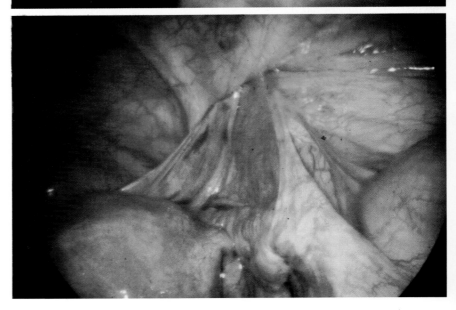

15.10 The effect of the traction is seen in this illustration.

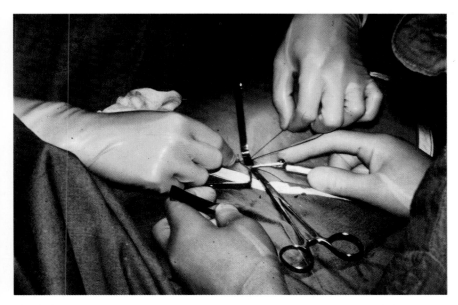

15.11 The round ligament is sutured to the rectus fascia.

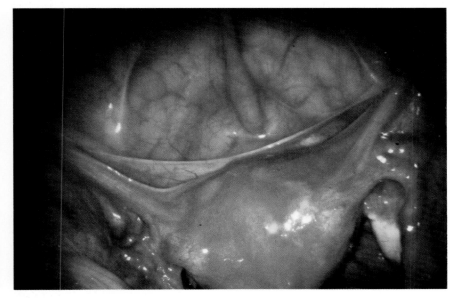

15.12 End result: The traction on the ligaments should not be excessive. It is the pressure of the abdominal contents that keeps the uterus in place.

Postoperative care

Hospitalization is longer than average—2 to 4 days. (Note from translator: In Europe as compared to the United States, hospitalization is usually longer by a factor of four.) During the first 2 weeks, suprapubic pain is quite common but easily treated with nonsteroidal anti-inflammatory agents.

Complications

The complications reported are rare and usually minor. Hematomas of the broad ligament, if stable, do not require any form of treatment. Resorption takes several days. These hematomas may lead to unilateral release of a suture, a rare but awful complication because it causes pain related to torsion of the uterus and requires reintervention. More severe complications, such as laceration of the epigastric or iliac vessels, can occur. A good knowledge of anatomy and technique will help to avoid such complications.

Indications

We agree with the majority of authors that retroversion should be corrected only if there are symptoms, in particular dyspareunia. Physical examination should reproduce this pain during vaginal and especially rectal examination.

Additional tests

Additional tests are not required, even if hysterophlebography (transuterine) and phlebography with radioisotopes [10] objectively demonstrate venous stasis associated with retroversion.

Indications

Laparoscopy allows differentiation between the types of retroversion. Secondary retroversion is due to obstetrical trauma or the presence of concomitant pathology.

Mobile retroversion

This is the most frequent type. It is due to breakdown of the uterine support during childbirth several months or years before, the time necessary for the symptoms to develop. Visual inspection of the pelvis reveals all the symptoms of venous engorgement previously described. The uterus is extremely mobile; frequently one or both uterosacral ligaments have disappeared. This is the syndrome described by Allen and Masters. The postoperative outcome depends on how well the uterus is supported and how strong the round ligaments are.

Fixed retroversion

Retroversion by a complex of adhesions is less frequent. There is additional pathology, which usually expresses itself in specific symptoms: previous pelvic inflammatory disease or surgery and, of course, endometriosis with obliteration of the cul-de-sac. Laparoscopy is the test of choice for evaluation of the pelvic pathology. Obviously, with regard to treatment, uterine suspension is of less importance than treatment of the primary pathology. However, if the dynamic tests show improvement of uterine vascularization, a suspension should be done. Moreover, this will avoid continued contact between the ovaries and the raw surfaces of the cul-de-sac.

Contraindications

Primary or congenital retroversion

This condition is generally asymptomatic and is probably related to a congenital weakness of the uterine support. It is often associated with hypoplasia of the uterus and is more a retroflexion than a retroversion. During laparoscopy, one can see a normally colored uterus, often hypoplastic, with ligaments (round and sacrouterine) that have a rudimentary aspect. The uterus typically shows a curvature of the anterior wall, as if the anterior wall had outgrown the posterior wall. There is no sign of venous stasis. Treatment of this condition is unnecessary and bound to fail.

Abnormal insertion of the round ligament

This apparently occurs more often than one would think. The round ligaments insert lower than normal toward the isthmus uteri. Suspension will bring the isthmus higher, but rarely will the corpus become anteverted beyond a vertical plane (in the upright position). Intra-abdominal pressure is likely to compromise the outcome.

False retroversions

These are less frequently encountered since the widespread use of sonography. Sometimes, however, the wrong diagnosis is uncovered at laparoscopy:
- Uterine myoma of the posterior wall
- Adnexal mass prolapsed in the cul-de-sac

Results

TABLE 15.1 **Laparoscopic uterine suspension**

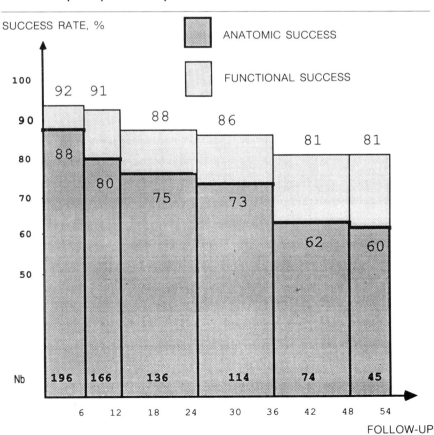

Table 15.1 shows the long-term results in terms of the stability of the uterine position and the recurrence of symptoms. Overall, the success rate is high and the effect persists, justifying a minor procedure. One should note that recurrence of retroversion is more frequent than recurrence of the symptoms. This is a well-known phenomenon due to unknown factors, possibly vascular or psychological. This type of discongruence is a phenomenon that occurs frequently in medicine, even when anatomic lesions are clearly observed. All other series report a similar phenomenon [1, 4, 6–8].

Anatomic correction was maintained during and after pregnancy in 11 out of a series of 16 patients. Other studies confirm this high incidence [3, 4, 6, 7, 8].

In conclusion, correction of retroversion by laparoscopy is simple, and this makes it the method of choice for treatment of chronic pelvic pain. Causes of chronic pelvic pain other than retroversion must be carefully investigated, however, including the psychological aspects, as all play a role.

References

1. Abeille J.P., « Cure de rétrodéviation per cœlioscopie, série de 35 cas », *Gynécologie*, 1975; 26 (6) : 437-441.
2. Abeille J.P., « Peut-on espérer traiter les rétroversions par cœlioscopie », *J. Gynecol. Obstet. Biol. Reprod.*, 1976; 5 : 723.
3. Bernard P., Sage J.C., Vignaud D.B., Debon J., « La ligamentopexie per-cœlioscopique », *Med. Prat.*, 1978; 2 : 62-69.
4. Brun G., Vandeweghe C., « La ligamentopexie per-cœlioscopique », *Bordeaux Méd.*, 1978; 11 (15) : 1357-1359.
5. Bussière M.F., « La ligamentopexie per-cœlioscopique », 1984. Thèse, Université de Clermont-Ferrand I, 1984.
6. Durand A., Abeille J.P., « La cure de rétrodéviation per-cœlioscopique six ans après », *Gynécologie*, 1979; 30 (3) : 275-278.
7. Paterson M.E.L., Jordan J.A., Logan-Edwards R., « A survey of 100 patients who had laparoscopic ventro-suspensions », *Br. J. Obstet. Gynecol.*, 1978; 85 (6) : 468-471.
8. Racinet C., Sarorius C., Salvat J., Nammanovici C., « La ligamentopexie per-cœlioscopique, un test thérapeutique dans les algies pelviennes chroniques? », *Rev. Fr. Gynecol. Obstet.*, 1983; 78 (1) : 1-6.
9. Steptoe P.C., « Laparoscopy in Gynaecology », Livingstone, London, Edinburgh, 1967, 76.
10. Veyre A., Mage G., Pauletto B., Bruhat M.A., « Hystérophlébographie isotopique », Symposium International sur la veine pelvienne. Clermont-Ferrand, le 27 mai 1981. *Rev. Fr. Gynecol. Obstet.*, 1982.

16

Ovarian cysts

Routine gynecologic examination permits the discovery of many adnexal tumors which, on ultrasonography, are shown to be cystic. It is still true that persistent cysts need to be thoroughly—and that means surgically—evaluated, because there is a chance of malignancy, even if both physical examination and ultrasonography are reassuring.

Introduction

Systematic laparotomy seems to us to be inappropriate because most of these lesions are benign and most patients young. Scars on the ovarian surface are known to develop adhesions easily [2, 4] and may therefore compromise future fertility. Moreover, at laparotomy, there is not enough information to opt for median versus Pfannenstiel incision.

Therefore, despite enormous progress in ultrasonography, laparoscopy is still extremely important for the diagnosis of adnexal masses and for choice of adequate, appropriate treatment. Whenever malignancy is suspected, a median laparotomy is performed. In the presence of a benign lesion, treatment can be performed under laparoscopic control.

This chapter condenses our experience in treating 508 adnexal cysts [13]. As a first step, only lesions considered to be benign, both clinically and ultrasonographically, are considered for laparoscopy. Ultrasonography, preferably transvaginal, is performed with extreme care, preferably by two physicians, if possible.

Procedure

Diagnosis (Figs. 16.1 through 16.11)

Inspection

Inspection is the first step and allows locating the tumor: ovarian, paraovarian, hydrosalpinx, or pseudoperitoneal cyst. In this chapter, we deal only with true ovarian cysts. Inspection of the ovary is aimed primarily at detecting papillary projections. Indeed, ultrasonography is ideal for detection of intracystic papillary structures, but it will miss extracystic lesions, because these are not surrounded by fluid.

A forceps introduced suprapubically is used to grasp the ovarian ligament for mobilization so that its entire surface can be inspected. The contralateral ovary, serosa, colic gutters, diaphragm, and liver are inspected equally carefully. Samples for cytology are obtained in all cases, either by aspiration or washings. The cystic or mixed cystic-solid nature of the ovary is evaluated by the degree of its translucence.

At this time two situations may arise:

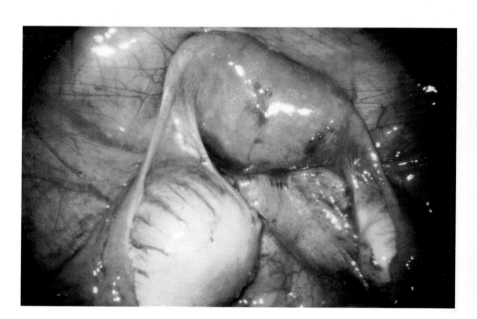

16.1 Organic ovarian cyst:
– comblike vascularization;
– elongated ovarian ligament.

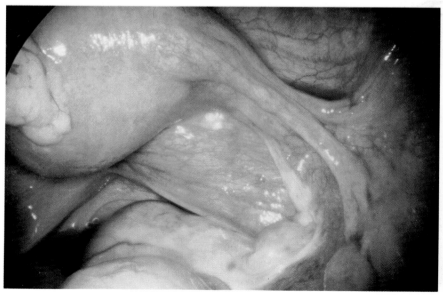

16.2 Organic ovarian cyst. There is significant elongation of the ovarian ligament (dermoid cyst).

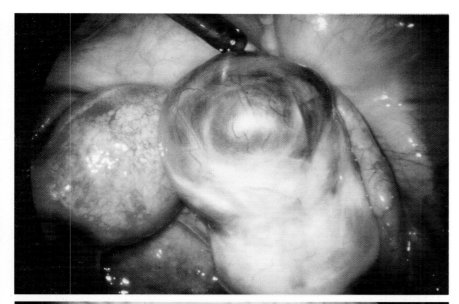

16.3 Two cysts on the right ovary:
– The front cyst (center of the figure) has the translucent wall and coraliform vascularization of a functional cyst.
– The other cyst shows the thick wall of an organic serous cystadenoma.

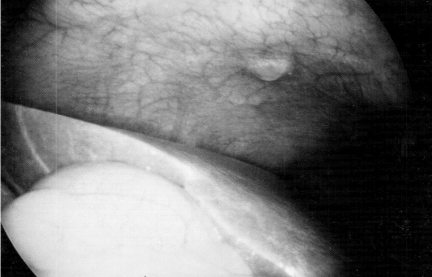

16.4 Inspection of the liver and diaphragm should be performed prior to puncture of the ovarian cyst.

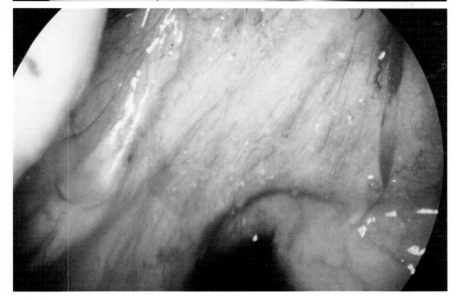

16.5 Micropapillae of the pelvic peritoneum.

– The tumor seems suspicious because of external papillary projections or because it appears more solid than cystic. A laparotomy is necessary. When the exophytic lesions are bright white, avascular, and hard, they may be no more than benign ovarian fibroids, to be confirmed by frozen section (Figs. 16.6, 16.7). Ovarian fibroids can be removed at laparoscopy. In all other cases, it is advisable to perform a laparotomy. Transparietal cystectomy following puncture of an ovarian cyst that appeared suspicious is a mistake because of the risk of metastasis in the abdominal wall, a situation we once witnessed.

– The tumor appears benign because the surface is smooth, regular, and of equal translucence. Puncture of the ovarian cyst then follows—the next step for diagnosis, but also for the first step in laparoscopic treatment.

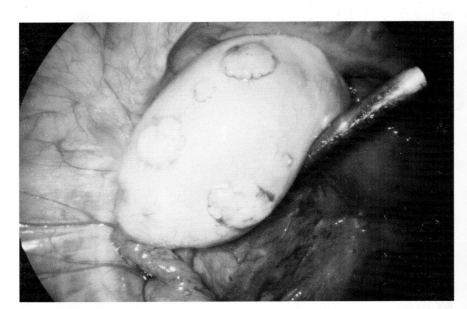

16.6 Benign growth of the ovary: papillary serous cystadenoma.

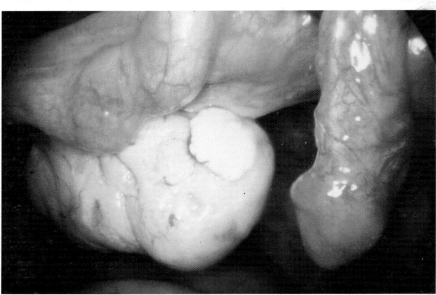

16.7 Benign growth of the ovary: fibrothecoma.

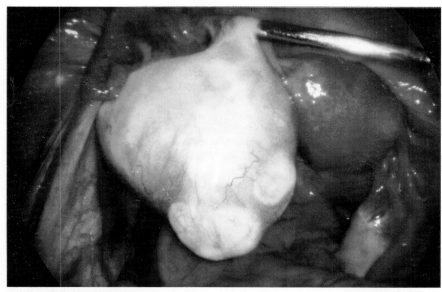

16.8 Mixed, cystic, and solid aspect of an ovarian cyst precludes puncture (histology = borderline tumor).

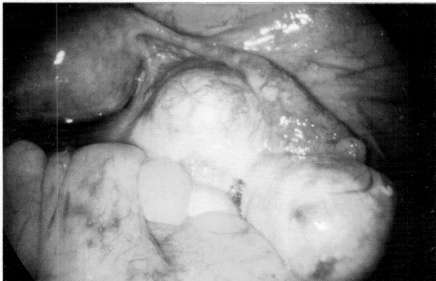

16.9 Another suspicious-looking ovarian cyst because of the irregular vascularization (histology = ovarian cancer).

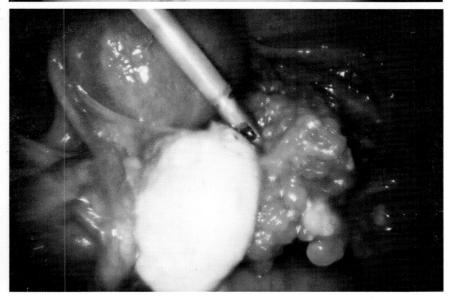

16.10 Exophytic lesions of the left ovary (mucinous cystadenoma). A laparotomy is indicated.

Puncture

This simple procedure can be done with a Verres needle or with a 5-mm trocar. The Verres needle is inserted through the abdominal wall immediately above the cyst. Aspiration is initiated prior to puncture of the cyst. In so doing, there will be minimal leakage. The 5-mm trocar is introduced suprapubically from the opposite side. The cyst is punctured and the trocar exchanged for an aspiration cannula (e.g., the Triton). The cyst is then evacuated and profusely rinsed. However, it is doubtful that intraperitoneal spillage can be avoided by either one of these techniques. Therefore it is mandatory to perform a complete peritoneal lavage after puncture of an ovarian cyst of which the diagnosis is unknown.

The macroscopic aspect of the cyst contents forms an integral part of the diagnosis. This aspect is different for each type of cyst (Table 16.1), and obviously the fluid, obtained prior to rinsing, must be sent for cytologic examination.

TABLE 16.1 **Diagnostic value of macroscopic appearance of the cyst fluid correlation with histologic diagnosis**

Histologic diagnosis	Cases		Fluid appearance					
			Clear	Yellow	Serohemorrhagic	Mucinous	Sebaceous	Chocolate
Functional	89	(96)[a]	11	49	26	1	—	2
Endometrioma	93	(100)	1	—	6	1	1	84
Serous	88	(100)	33	41	12	1	—	1
Mucinous	46	(51)	4	12	1	28	1	—
Teratoma	79	(91)	2	—	1	—	76	—
Borderline	1	(5)	—	—	1	—	—	—
Cancer	1	(4)	—	1	—	—	—	—
Paraovarian	55	(61)	44	7	3	1	—	—
Total	452	(508)	95	110	50	32	78	87

[a] Macroscopic appearance of the cyst fluid was not available in all cases (represented by numbers in parentheses).

Ovarian cystoscopy (Figs. 16.11 and 16.13)

Once emptied, the cyst is incised with scissors. The inner walls are inspected with the laparoscope in seach of papillary excrescences, which would lead to immediate laparotomy. At this stage, the surgeon should have enough information to classify the cyst as "probably benign," "functional," or "malignant" (Table 16.2). Table 16.3 summarizes the various criteria that allow differentiation between a functional and an organic cyst. These criteria are important, because they mandate a different therapeutic approach (see further).

TABLE 16.2 **Correlation between macroscopic appearance and histology**

Endoscopic appearance	Number of cases	Histology	
		Benign	Malignant or borderline
Benign	489	489	0
Malignant or suspicious	19	10	9
Total	508	499	9

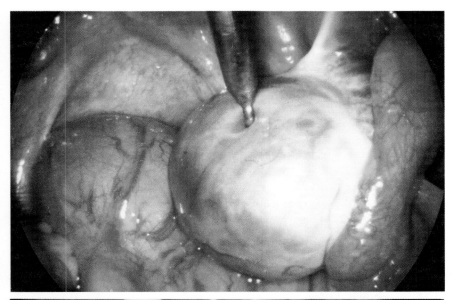

16.11 A functional cyst is characterized by a thin wall, absence of vessels, and a saffron-colored liquid.

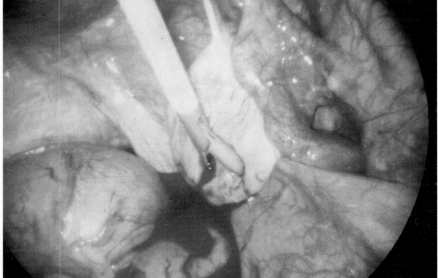

16.12 A biopsy is taken from the functional cyst.

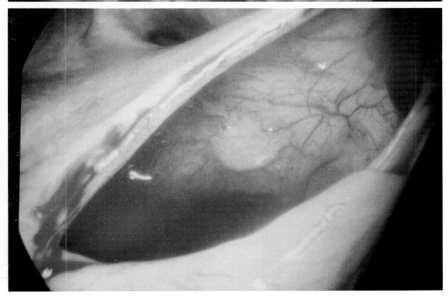

16.13 Typical retinoid aspect of the inside wall of a functional cyst.

Treatment

This discussion applies only to cysts that are considered benign or functional.

Puncture-biopsy (Fig. 16.12)

Puncture and puncture-biopsy of the cyst wall have the enormous disadvantage that the entire cyst wall is not available for diagnostic evaluation. This is therefore satisfactory only in the case of purely functional cysts. In case of doubt, cystectomy is preferable to avoid recurrence of an organic cyst or missing a diagnosis of malignancy.

Cystectomy

The objective is to excise the entire cyst wall. Indeed, many cysts are heterogenous, and only histologic examination of the entire cyst wall can reliably exclude malignancy. Moreover, this is the only conservative approach that will avoid recurrence.

Transparietal cystectomy (TPC) (Figs. 16.14 through 16.17)

This is a simple technique based on a minilaparotomy under laparoscopic control for resection of the cyst wall:

- Transverse incision of the skin (20 to 30 mm) in the midline or at the level of the cyst on a projected Pfannenstiel. The fascia is also incised transversely, and the muscle bluntly separated.
- Insertion of a forceps (Bengolea or curved Kelly) to grasp the ovary as far away from the hilus as possible (cyst punctured previously).
- Loss of pneumoperitoneum and extraction of ovary.
- Incision of peritoneum cranially and caudally to expose most of the ovary. It is important to incise the peritoneum at that time. The incision into the peritoneum must be long enough to facilitate reinsertion of the ovary into the abdomen after cystectomy.
- Incision of the ovarian cortex and extraction of the cyst wall as performed at laparotomy. The ovary is closed in two layers with Vicryl 4/0 or 6/0. Sometimes it is possible to omit suturing or to place only the deep sutures.
- Replacement of the ovary into the abdominal cavity, check of hemostasis, closure of the wall in three layers, and profuse rinsing-aspiration of the pelvic cavity.

The postoperative care is similar to that for any therapeutic laparoscopy. Hospitalization lasts 24 to 48 h. (Note from translator: In Europe, hospitalization is, on the average, four times longer than in the United States.)

Three comments must be made:

- Dermoid cysts usually cannot be emptied by aspiration prior to exteriorization because of the low suction pressure of the laparoscopic equipment.
- Extensive ovarian adhesions make the TPC approach impossible.
- Obesity limits the applicability of this technique.

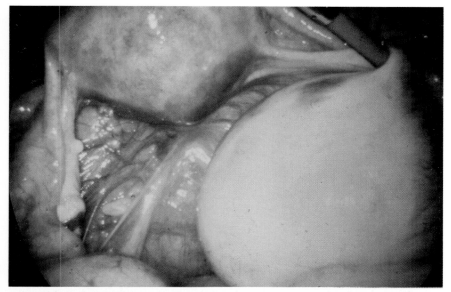

16.14 Benign organic cyst of the right ovary.

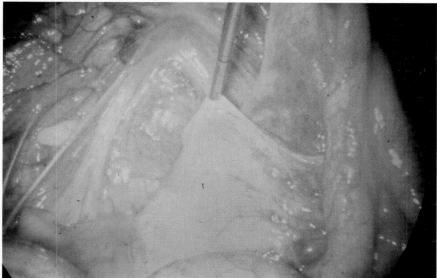

16.15 TPC: Puncture of the cyst.

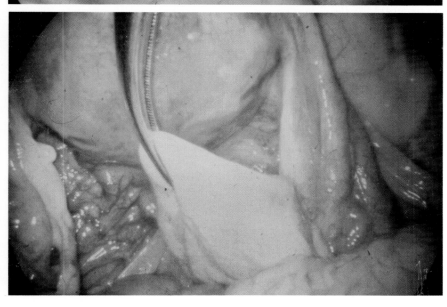

16.16 TPC: The cyst is grasped with a Kelly forceps after a 2 to 3 cm incision is made in the abdominal wall.

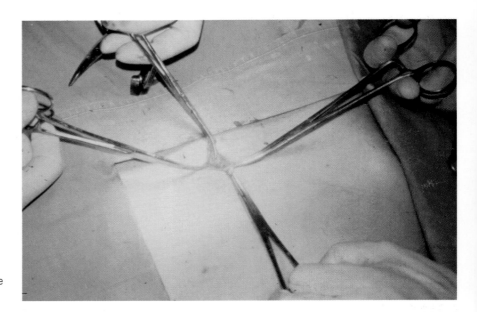

16.17 TPC: Classic cystectomy. Closure of the ovarian capsule is not mandatory.

Intraperitoneal (percutaneous) cystectomy (IPC) (Figs. 16.18 through 16.24)

Intraperitoneal (percutaneous) cystectomy is technically more difficult than TPC because the ovary is so mobile. Two variations are possible:

 - Puncture and opening of the cyst. The cyst wall is identified and, by traction, bluntly removed from its ovarian bed. Dissection is done carefully, repositioning the forceps regularly as close to the cleavage plane as possible. It is often more effective to peel off the ovarian cortex than to pull on the cyst. Once resected, the cyst is removed through the trocar. Hemostasis is rarely required. If necessary, POR 8 can be injected into the mesoovary. This technique is effective for small serous cysts.

 - Incision of the ovarian cortex only, before puncture. Cleavage of the cyst off the ovary is obtained by blunt dissection, and puncture is done at the end of the procedure. This technique applies to cysts which one is sure are benign, such as paraovarian cysts. Indeed, previous puncture makes blunt dissection of these cysts more difficult.

Hospitalization lasts 24 to 48 h.

Endosurgical oophorectomy

This procedure was described by Semm, using Roeder loops and the morcellator for removal of the ovary. This appears to us to be of only limited value. The main advantage of laparoscopy is its conservative nature. Indications for oophorectomy are rare unless there is suspicion of malignancy, which, in our opinion, excludes the use of an instrument such as the morcellator. Oophorectomy, although rarely indicated, can be achieved using the IPC approach.

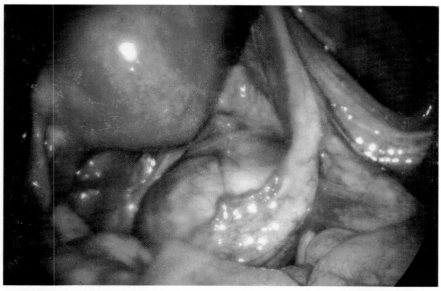

16.18   Right paraovarian cyst.

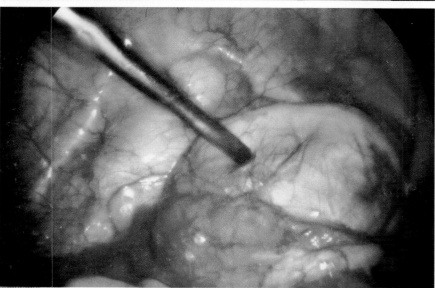

16.19   IPC: Puncture of the cyst.

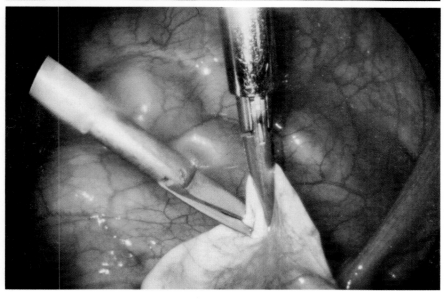

16.20   IPC: Opening of the cyst.

16.21–16.23 IPC: Blunt dissection of the cyst wall by traction with two forceps.

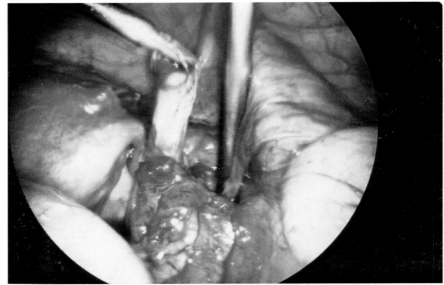

16.21

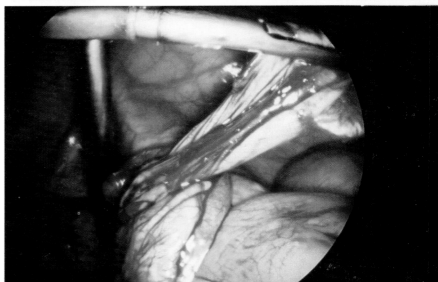

16.22

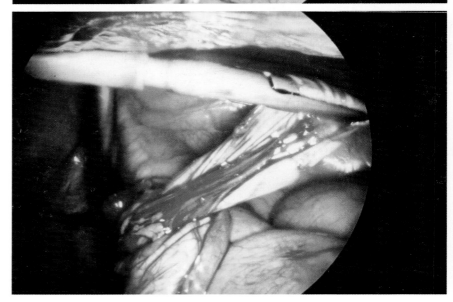

16.23

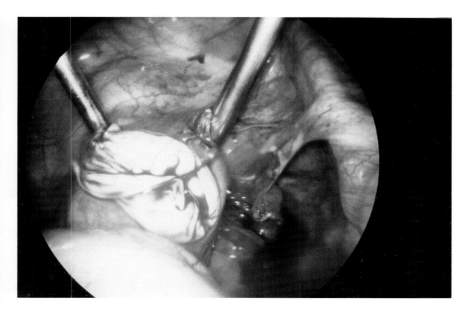

16.24 IPC: End result.

Indications

Laparoscopy is important for diagnosis of lesions, especially to rule out hydrosalpinx, pseudoperitoneal cysts, etc., complementing information given by ultrasonography which, in fact, can be difficult to interpret in the presence of multiple adhesions. At the time of laparoscopy, a decision for further treatment can be made.

Paraovarian cysts

This type of cyst highlights the value of laparoscopy because, clinically and ultrasonographically, they are indistinguishable from ovarian cysts. Moreover, treatment by IPC is quite easy.

Ovarian cysts

Laparoscopy is the end point of a well-defined clinical investigation.
   - The initial physical examination is followed by ultrasonography of the pelvis and radiography of the abdomen.
   - Cystic tumors of less than 8 cm are treated with oral contraception with 50 μg ethinyl estradiol daily for 3 months, then reevaluated.
   - Patients with persistent cystic masses are scheduled for laparoscopy.
   - In all other cases, patients are hospitalized for exploratory laparotomy if malignancy is suspected. A laparoscopy is performed in case of doubt.
   The endoscopic procedure is performed as described above. Puncture of the ovarian cyst is allowed in the absence of any indication of malignancy. In a 7-year period of time, 481 patients (508 cysts) were evaluated via laparoscopy. We use these data to estimate the accuracy of laparoscopy in the diagnosis of malignancy and in diagnosis of the type of organic (benign) cyst.

Diagnosis of malignancy (Table 16.2)

In our series, not a single malignant or borderline tumor was missed. On the other hand, 10 cysts thought to be malignant were revealed to be benign. When the cyst was described as benign, this was confirmed by histologic examination in all cases. These results deserve some comment:

– The number of malignant tumors is small, and these results will have to be confirmed. Of the 9 tumors, 7 were of stage I and the 2 others stage III, with small total tumor mass; therefore all these tumors have a good prognosis.

– The high incidence of false-positive evaluation of malignancy is not a negative factor, in our opinion. It reflects the caution of the surgeons, an essential element in the treatment of ovarian lesions.

– Finally, it must be emphasized that the suspicion of malignancy preceded puncture of the lesion in 7 out of 9 patients. Thus, in our hands, the puncturing of lesions seems to bear only a low risk of spreading cancer cells. Moreover, all cysts evaluated as being benign were confirmed as such on histologic examination.

One must, however, consider the problems that could arise from puncture of an ovarian malignancy even if puncture does not equal rupture so far as the spread of cells is concerned. When one deals with a borderline tumor [9, 10, 24], rupture does not seem to influence the spread of the disease provided the tumor is removed immediately. When dealing with ovarian cancer, the data in the literature are divergent. Some authors do not consider rupture to have a negative impact on prognosis [3, 8, 19, 23]; others do [11, 14, 25]. Two reasons may explain this apparent contradiction. First of all, accidental rupture of tumors probably occurs more often when the mass is large and adherent to surrounding structures. These adhesions may be reactions to spontaneous "leaks" of the tumor, which is a different situation from rupture resulting from surgical manipulation. Second, staging of the tumors in these studies was often incomplete, so that it is not warranted to compare groups under these circumstances. Nonetheless, such studies are scarce and as long as there is no definitive answer as to what effect puncture has, it should be performed with caution.

Finally, one should balance the theoretical risk of puncture of an ovarian cancer against the true benefit of early diagnosis by minimally invasive surgery. Also, patients more readily accept the necessity to undergo laparoscopy than laparotomy for investigation of a cyst that is asymptomatic most of the time.

Diagnosis of benign cysts

It is important to differentiate organic cysts from functional cysts, either found incidentally or persisting under hormonal suppression. Simple puncture of an organic cyst leads to recurrence. Table 16.3 summarizes the five stages which allow differentiation.

When in doubt, the high concentration of estradiol in functional cysts is helpful. Tables 16.4 and 16.5 summarize the results of our series.

The most frequent error is mistaking small serous cystadenomas and paraovarian cysts for functional cysts. To minimize the possibility of leaving an organic cyst untreated, an attempt at cystectomy should always be made.

Benign organic cysts

The diagnosis of the exact nature of the cyst is less critical because the entire cyst will have to be removed in any case. However, for the surgical procedure, it may be important to know more specifically what kind of cyst one is dealing with.

– *Serous cystadenoma:* A rounded, unilocular, smooth tumor with a dough-like consistency. The cyst wall is pearly white or sometimes bluish. The vessels are regularly disposed ("comblike"). The fluid is mostly clear, sometimes yellowish, and rarely hemorrhagic.

TABLE 16.3 **Endoscopic differentiation of ovarian cysts**

	Functional cyst	Organic cyst
Ovarian ligament	Normal length	Elongated
Cyst wall	Thin	Thick
Vascularization	Coralliform, abundant	Comblike, poorly developed
Fluid	Saffron yellow, hemorrhagic	Variable, according to histologic type
Inner surface of cyst wall	Retinoid	Smooth or papillary

TABLE 16.4 **Correlation with histologic diagnosis**

Endoscopic appearance	Number of cases	Histologic diagnosis			
		Functional	Organic	Borderline	Cancer
Functional	93	83	10	—	—
Organic					
Benign	396	13	383	—	—
Suspicious	14	—	10	4	—
Cancer	5	—	—	1	4
Total	508	96	403	5	4

TABLE 16.5 **Correlation between macroscopic diagnosis by laparoscopy and definitive pathologic diagnosis**

Macroscopic laparoscopic diagnosis	Definitive pathologic diagnosis								
	Cases	Functional	Endometrioma	Serous	Mucinous	Teratoma	Borderline	Cancer	Paraovarian
Functional	93	83	3	6	—	—	—	—	1
Endometrioma	102	6	93	2	—	1	—	—	—
Serous	99	6	1	79	11	1	—	—	1
Mucinous	40	—	—	2	38	—	—	—	—
Teratoma	92	—	2	1	1	88	—	—	—
Suspicious	14	—	1	7	1	1	4	—	—
Cancer	5	—	—	—	—	—	1	4	—
Paraovarian	63	1	—	3	—	—	—	—	59
Total	508	96	100	100	51	91	5	4	61

— *Mucinous cystadenoma:* An often multiloculated tumor that is bluish or grayish in color. The vascularization is somewhat more pronounced than with serous cystadenoma. The fluid is clear and viscous—quite characteristic when sufficient fluid is present. In smaller cysts, the viscosity of the fluid is less obvious.

— *Dermoid cyst:* Unilocular with a thick, white wall having yellow patches. The ovary is extremely heavy. The fluid contains sebaceous grease and hair.

— *Endometriotic cyst:* Identified thanks to the surrounding peritoneal lesions and to the brown deposits on the ovarian surfaces. The endometriotic cyst has a relatively poor vascular supply. Chocolate-type fluid is pathognomonic, but it can be quite thin and consequently difficult to differentiate from the fluid of a hemorrhagic corpus luteum.

The most common mistake involves small mucinous cystadenomas being mistaken for serous cystadenomas, which is of no consequence.

Only systematic biopsy will solve the confusion between functional cysts and endometriomas. Fortunately, the consequences are limited because puncture biopsy followed by medical treatment of the endometrioma may very well give good results.

Results: Efficiency of laparoscopic treatment

Among 481 patients (508 cysts) undergoing surgical exploration for adnexal mass, 420 (87.4 %) (444 cysts) were treated via laparoscopy. The 61 laparotomies were performed for the following reasons: suspicion of malignancy (19 cases) and large cysts (42 cases) (Table 16.6). Of the 444 cysts treated by laparoscopy, 412 (92.8 %) conservative treatments, 32 oophorectomies, and 1 adnectomy were performed. These data are summarized in Tables 16.7 and 16.8. Not a single postoperative hemorrhage occurred. Hospitalization lasted 2 to 3 days. Postoperative course was uncomplicated in all but 3 cases. One case of acute abdominal pain underwent a second laparoscopy, which failed to show any pathology. Two cases of ovarian abscess were diagnosed 4 weeks after intervention; these were treated conservatively, one by laparoscopy and the other by laparotomy. In all, 230 patients have been followed for 1 to 6 years with no recurrence (excluding endometriomas).

It is important to discuss puncture and opening of dermoid and mucinous cysts.

– Rupture of a mucinous cystadenoma can theoretically lead to pseudomyxoma peritonei. However, this disease usually involves the entire peritoneum at the time of first presentation [9, 22] and very often is associated with a cystadenocarcinoma [6, 12, 17]. Rupture of cystadenocarcinoma rarely leads to pseudomyxoma [9]. We have never observed pseudomyxoma after treatment of mucinous cystadenoma by laparoscopy.

– Peritoneal granulomatosis is a rare complication of dermoid cysts. We have not observed this in our series. A few cases have been described after puncture during laparoscopy or ultrasonography [5, 15, 18, 21], but there was a delay of 3 to 12 weeks between puncture and excision. Immediate removal seems to avoid this complication [7]. Systematic surgical exploration of the contralateral ovary has become obsolete since the advent of ultrasonography, which is able to detect bilateral lesions.

In all cases, and especially when dealing with mucinous or dermoid cysts, puncture should be as watertight as possible, followed by excision and careful rinsing of the pelvis in one session. Recurrence after simple puncture is estimated to be 25 % [16]. We therefore advocate total excision of the cyst wall.

Conclusion

There are 10 requirements that must be fulfilled before conservative treatment of a cyst can be initiated.

TABLE 16.6 **Treatment of 481 patients**

```
481 patients → 508 cysts
   447 ovarian cysts (88 %)
     96 functional cysts (21.5 %)
    351 organic ovarian cysts (78.5 %)
     61 paraovarian cysts (12 %)
Managed by laparotomy
     61 patients (12.6 %) → 64 cysts
     19 malignant or suspicious
     42 dense adhesion or large cysts
Managed by laparoscopy
    420 patients (87.4 %) → 444 cysts
     95 functional cysts
     58 paraovarian cysts
    291 organic ovarian cysts
```

TABLE 16.7 **Laparoscopic management of adnexal cystic tumors according to pathologic diagnosis**

Definitive pathologic diagnosis	Cases	Treatment			
		Laparoscopic treatment		Laparotomy	
		N	%	N	%
Functional	96	95	99	1	1
Low malignancy potential and cancer	9	0	0	9	100
Benign organic ovarian cysts	342	291	85.08	51	14.9
Parovarian	61	58	95.1	3	4.9

TABLE 16.8 **Laparoscopic management of adnexal cystic tumors according to pathologic diagnosis**

Definitive pathologic diagnosis	Cases	Laparoscopic treatment		TPC		IPC		Oophorectomy		Puncture biopsy		Laser vaporization	
		N	%	N	%	N	%	N	%	N	%	N	%
Functional	96	95	99	9	9.4	16	16.7	1	1	69	71.9		
Borderline and cancer	9	0	0	0									
Paraovarian	61	58	95.1	12	19.7	43	70.5			3	4.9		
Endometrioma	100	90	90	8	8	50	50	1	1	25	25	6	6.6
Serous	100	87	87	29	29	39	39	14	14	5	5		
Mucinous	51	45	88.2	19	37.3	21	41.2	5	9.8				
Teratoma	91	78	85.7	32	35.2	26	28.6	11	12.1				

1) No clinical signs of malignancy

2) No echographical signs of malignancy

3) No laparoscopic signs of malignancy (extracystic papillary projections, negative exploration of the abdomen)

4) Systematic sampling of the peritoneal fluid for cytology

5) Cystoscopy for detection of intracystic papillary structures, which should lead to exploratory laparotomy

6) Puncture valid only if followed by biopsy and only when dealing with a functional cyst

7) Exploration, with puncture, if necessary, of the contralateral ovary

8) Profuse rinsing-aspiration of peritoneal cavity at the end of the procedure

9) Anatomopathology to include

- Cytology of peritoneal fluid
- Cytology of cyst fluid
- Histology of cyst wall

10) Follow-up with serial ultrasonographic and clinical examination

References

1. Abeille J.P., Moing M.H., Legros R., Scholler R., Castanier M., Nahoul K., « Le corps jaune kystique: un aspect cœlioscopique particulier de la pathologie fonctionnelle ovarienne. Confrontations laparo-biologiques », *Rev. Fr. Gynecol. Obstet.*, 1978; 73 : 19-27.

2. Buttram V.C., Vaquero C., « Post-ovarian wedge resection adhesive disease », *Fertil. Steril.*, 1975; 26 : 874.

3. Dembo A.J., « Radiation therapy in the management of ovarian cancer », *Clin. Obstet. Gynaecol.*, 1983; 10 : 261.

4. Donnez J., « Facteurs étiologiques de la stérilité tubaire », *J. Gynecol. Obstet. Biol. Reprod.*, 1983; 12 : 451.

5. Dorangeon P., Palmer R., « L'intérêt de la cœlioscopie dans le dépistage des tumeurs malignes de l'ovaire », *Bull. Fed. Gynecol. Obstet.*, 1963; 15 : 301.

6. Fernandez R.N., Daly J.M., « Pseudomyxoma Peritonaei », *Arch. Surg.*, 1980; 115 : 409.

7. Frangenheim H., Stockhammer H., « La laparoscopie dans le diagnostic différentiel des tumeurs du petit bassin chez les femmes ménopausées », *Gynécologie*, 1969; 167 : 503-510.

8. Grogan R.H., « Accidental rupture of malignant ovarian cysts during surgical removal », *Obstet. Gynecol.*, 1967; 30 : 716.

9. Hart W.R., Norris H.J., « Borderline and malignant mucinous tumors of the ovary », *Cancer*, 1973; 31 : 1031.

10. Hopkins M.P., Kumar N.B., Morley C.W., « An assessment of pathologic and treatment modalities in ovarian tumors of low malignant potential », *Obstet. Gynecol.*, 1987; 70 : 923.

11. Hsiu J.G., Given F.T., Kemp G.M., « Tumor implantation after diagnostic laparoscopic biopsy of serous ovarian tumors of low malignant potential », *Obstet. Gynecol.*, 1986; 68 : 905.

12. Limber G.K., King R.E., Silverberg S.G., « Pseudomyxoma Peritonei: a report of ten cases », *Ann. Surg.*, 1973; 178 : 587.

13. Mage G., Canis M., Manhes H., Pouly J.L., Bruhat M.A., « Kystes ovariens et cœlioscopie », *J. Gynecol. Obstet. Biol. Reprod.*, 1987; 16 : 1053-1061.

14. Malkasian G.D., Melton L.J., O'Brien P.C., Greene M.H., « Prognostic significance of histologic classification and grading of epithelial malignancies of the ovary », *Am. J. Obstet. Gynecol.*, 1984; 149 : 274.

15. Mintz M., de Brux J., « La ponction per-cœlioscopique et la cytologie de 307 kystes intra-pelviens. Etude critique de ses indications diagnostiques et thérapeutiques », *Gynécologie*, 1974; 25 : 63-74.

16. Mintz M., Bessis R., Brodaty C., Pez J.P., « Que deviennent les kystes para-utérins ponctionnés sous cœlioscopie? Apports de l'échographie », *Gynécologie*, 1983; 34 : 451-463.

17. Novetsky S., Berlin L., Epstein J., « Pseudomyxoma Peritonei », *J. Comput. Assist. Tomogr.*, 1982; 6 : 398.

18. Peterson W.F., « Malignant degeneration of benign cystic teratomas of the ovary. Collective revue of the literature », *Obstet. Gynecol. Surg.*, 1957; 12: 793.

19. Purola E., Nieminen U., « Does rupture of cystic carcinoma during operation influence prognosis? », *Ann. Chir. Gynaecol. Fenniae*, 1968; 57 : 615-617.

20. Randall C.D., Hall D.W., « Clinical consideration of benign ovarian cystadenomas », *Am. J. Obstet. Gynecol.*, 1951; 62 : 806.

21. Ranney B., Facog M.D., « Iatrogenic spillage from benign ovarian cystomas », *Am. J. Obstet. Gynecol.*, 1951; 62 : 806-815.

22. Scully R.E., « Common epithelial tumors of borderline malignancy (carcinomas of low malignant potential », *Bull. Cancer*, 1982; 69 : 228.

23. Sigurdsson K., Alm P., Gullberg B., « Prognostic factors in malignant epithelial ovarian tumors », *Gynecol. Oncol.*, 1983; 15 : 370.

24. Tasker M., Langley F.A., « The outlook for women with borderline epithelial tumors of the ovary », *Br. J. Obstet. Gynecol.*, 1985; 92 : 969.

25. Webb M.J., Decker D.G., Mussey E., Williams T.J., « Factors influencing survival in Stage I ovarian cancer », *Am. J. Obstet. Gynecol.*, 1973; 116 : 222.

17

Adnexal torsion

Torsion is defined as rotation of part or all of the adnexa around an axis, leading to vascular obstruction, partial or complete—an emergency situation [1]. The degree of rotation is usually greater than 360°. Some ischemic lesions have been reported in association with a rotation of only 110° [2]. Torsion involving malignant lesions and chronic torsion secondary to adhesions or due to endometriosis are excluded from the series presented.

Pathophysiology

Incidence

Adnexal torsion is rare. We observed 38 cases in more than 10,000 laparoscopies. It occurs in women of reproductive age [1–4], and bilateral lesions are truly exceptional (16 cases reported) [5].

Clinical presentation

Two scenarios are possible (Table 17.1):
- Acute torsion where absence of prodromal signs makes diagnosis difficult.
- Chronic torsion discovered at the time of diagnostic laparoscopy for adnexal mass.

In both cases, diagnosis requires surgical exploration. Laparoscopy therefore eliminates unnecessary laparotomy in acute forms (ectopic, bleeding corpus luteum) as well as in chronic forms (paratubal cysts, persistent corpus luteum) and allows conservative treatment in a large proportion (63.4 %) of cases.

TABLE 17.1 **Adnexal torsion**

Clinical presentation	Number of cases	Extent of lesions		
		Minimal	Severe	Irreversible necrosis
Acute	29	15	8	6
Chronic	9	9	0	0
Total	38	24	8	6

Diagnosis

Laparoscopy leaves little doubt about the diagnosis. It is then important to evaluate the affected organs: tube, ovary or both, their pathology, and the degree of ischemia. This information is essential to making the choice between radical or conservative treatment. Conservative treatment using laparoscopy is done when one estimates that the ischemia is reversible and that the pathology presented can be treated via laparoscopy (24 of 38 cases; 63.4 %).

Procedure

Surgical conservative treatment encompasses detorsion and treatment of the etiology. Detorsion also allows recognition of the contraindications to conservative surgery.

Detorsion (Figs. 17.1 through 17.6)

Detorsion is easily performed with a blunt probe or an atraumatic forceps. One should:
   – Recognize the direction of rotation of the adnexa, keeping in mind the law of Kustner, which states that the adnexa always rotate *toward* the uterus clockwise for the left adnexa and *counterclockwise* for the right.
   – Bluntly mobilize rather than grasp the adnexa.
   – Progressively return the adnexa to a normal anatomic position.
A second probe may be necessary to stabilize the organs during detorsion. Detorsion is easier when the volume of the adnexa is small, thus initial puncture of, for example, a paraovarian cyst is helpful. In some cases, transection of a bride or pedicle from a hydatid cyst is followed by spontaneous detorsion. We are convinced that detorsion is required because the operator should be able to evaluate how well the adnexa recuperates. During the initial phase of reopening of the vessels, Way [18] advocates the use of warm gauze on the adnexa. At laparoscopy, one can introduce 500 mL of warm physiologic saline into the cul-de-sac. In a retrospective study of 38 cases, we have catalogued the lesions as follows (Table 17.1):
   – Mild degree: The congestion of the adnexa disappears shortly after detorsion. The ovary is increased in volume and edematous and the tube is congested but of normal volume.
   – Severe degree: The tube is dark red or even purple. The organs under torsion are extremely distended. After detorsion, the tube recuperates relatively quickly, the ovary much more slowly. Observation of a normal-appearing cortex around the hilus is an excellent prognostic sign.
   – Irreversible torsion: The adnexa is black, friable, extremely enlarged, and sometimes covered with a fibrinous exudate. Detorsion brings no improvement and sometimes the adnexa abrupt during the maneuver. Irreversible torsion is uncommon (6 in 38 cases = 15.7 %) and is a complication that can be prevented by early diagnosis and treatment.

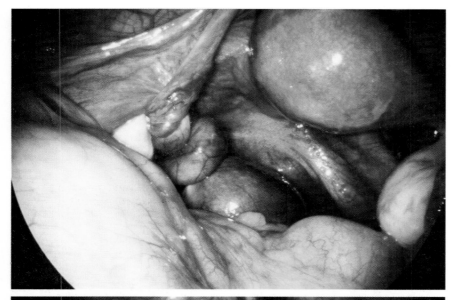

17.1 Torsion of the left oviduct, caused by a para-ovarian cyst. There are three rotations and minimal ischemia.

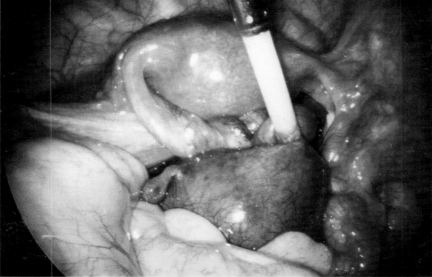

17.2–17.4 Mobilization of the tube with a blunt probe causes detorsion. This surgical maneuver should be slow and gentle because of the delicacy of the tissues.

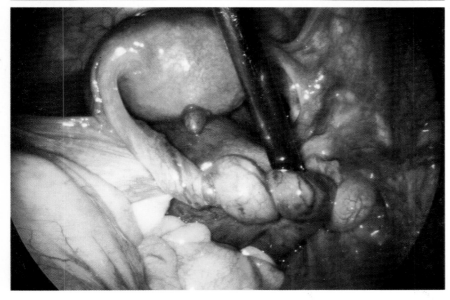

17.3

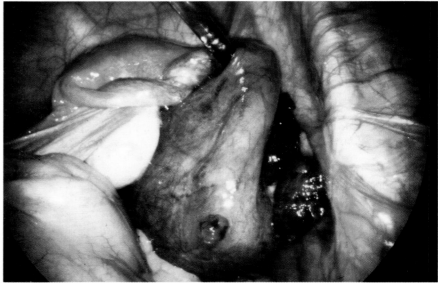

17.4

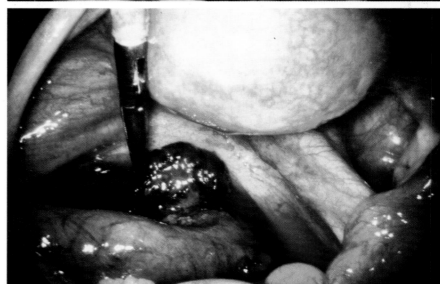

17.5 Aspect of the tube at completion of surgery.

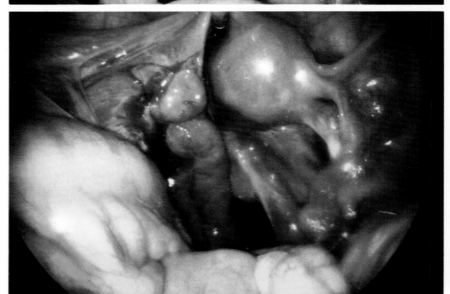

17.6 End result: the paraovarian cyst has been removed. The incision into the mesosalpinx was made lateral to the tube. The oviduct has a nearly normal appearance.

Conservative treatment versus radical treatment

The appearance of the adnexa guides the choice:
  − Irreversible necrosis of the organs mandates surgical excision.
  − Mild lesions may be treated conservatively if etiologic factors permit.
  − Severe lesions (Figs. 17.7 through 17.11) will benefit from a conservative approach, despite the initial aspect of the adnexa. This approach calls for systematic insertion of a drain and hospitalization for 4 to 5 days. (Note from translator: In Europe, hospitalization is, on the average, four times longer than in the United States.) In a series of 8 second-look laparoscopies at 6 to 8 weeks after detorsion, all cases showed complete recovery, which confirms the value of the conservative approach, as observed by Way [18].

  • Conservative management has been challenged by many authors [2, 4]. Indeed, detorsion has been heavily criticized for fear of embolism [2, 4]. We observed no complications related to possible embolism, nor did Way in a series of 15 patients, including severe cases, nor did MacGowan and Lomano, reporting on mild cases [18, 12, 11].
  • Anatomic regeneration remains a source of wonder, both histologically and functionally.
    − One of our patients with only one adnexa, treated for torsion approximately 72 h after onset of symptoms (Figs. 17.1, 17.2, 17.3) had a normal intrauterine pregnancy 8 months later. Before that an ovarian biopsy taken at second-look laparoscopy revealed a normal concentration of follicles.
    − Tubal patency has been demonstrated with hysterosalpingography after conservative treatment [1, 6].
    − Hurwitz reported on normal progress of a pregnancy after conservative treatment of a torsed luteal cyst [8]. Two of our patients were diagnosed and treated in the second month of pregnancy and did well.
    − The tolerance of the ovary to prolonged ischemia is remakable, as has been demonstrated by animal research. An ovary transplanted without its pedicle in the rabbit will remain functional up to 25 days [10].

These arguments are admittedly anecdotal, but in our opinion adequate to advocate conservative management of severe cases in every young female.

Many factors affect the severity of ischemic lesions:
  − The duration of the torsion is the most important element. The interval between initial pain and diagnosis was always longer than 72 h in severe cases.
  − The number of turns (four or more lead to severe torsion).
  − The volume of the adnexa, by pulling on the pedicle, worsens the vascular obstruction.

Second-look laparoscopy should be routine, even in uncomplicated cases. Indeed, it is difficult to evaluate with accuracy the severity of the ischemia and its evolution.

A second-look also allows an anatomic and functional assessment. The examination of the ovary at the time of detorsion may not have been accurate if the lesion was small. A more accurate evaluation can be made at second-look laparoscopy. Follow-up of ovarian cysts can be done with the help of serial ultrasonography.

Detorsion is a necessary step in conservative management of torsion. The risk for thromboembolic accident has thus far remained more theoretical than real.

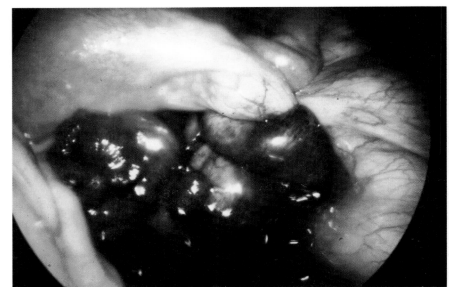

17.7 Severe ischemia of single adnexa, resulting from 72 h of torsion without apparent etiology.

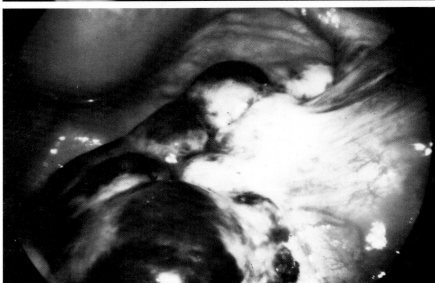

17.8 Aspect of the tube after detorsion. The ovarian tissue close to the mesentery shows a nearly normal coloration.

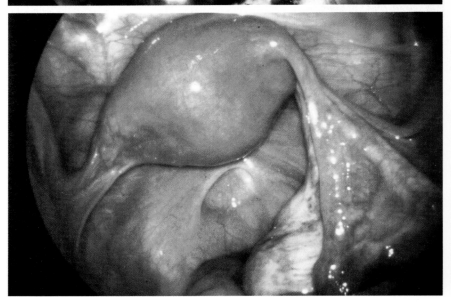

17.9 Follow-up laparoscopy in the same patient as in Figs. 17.7 and 17.8, two months after the torsion. A biopsy shows a normal concentration of primordial follicles.

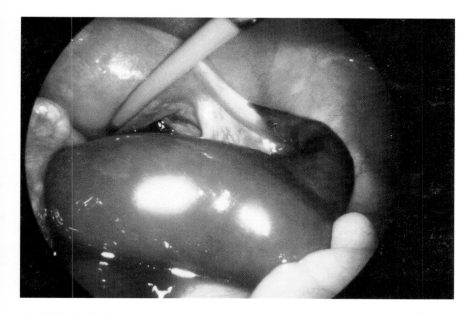

17.10 Appearance of an oviduct after detorsion. No lesion could be detected. The patient was young, so an ectopic pregnancy was highly unlikely.

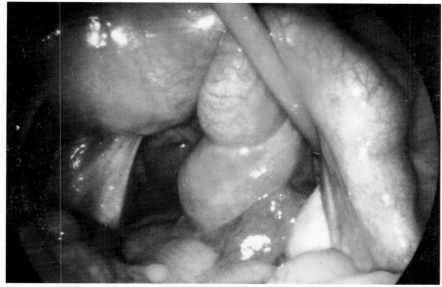

17.11 The same as in Fig. 17.10. Convalescence was astonishing, and the oviduct is patent. The global aspect, however, indicates that the acute torsion led to some sequelae.

Diagnosing and treating the cause of torsion

Different etiologies call for different treatments. Table 17.2 classifies the lesions observed in the 38 patients treated in our department. The techniques actually used for treatment of the various conditions are discussed in their respective chapters.

Torsion of the normal adnexa [14, 15]

Reported in many series, this is a diagnosis made by exclusion. Three requirements ought to be fulfilled before one accepts the diagnosis of normal ovary:
  - Multiple punctures of the ovary have excluded the presence of a small cyst.
  - Detorsion is stable. An immediate return to the torsed position evokes the possibility of abnormality and the necessity of ovariopexy.
  - Inspection of the tube reveals no pathology such as an ectopic pregnancy.

TABLE 17.2 **Adnexal torsion**

Etiologic factor	Organs involved			
	Tube	Ovary	Adnexa	Total
Paraovarian cyst	6		7	12
Functional ovarian cyst			5[a]	5[a]
Organic ovarian cyst			9	9
Ectopic pregnancy	2			2
Adhesions	2		1[a]	3[a]
Congenital malformation		1	1	2
Normal anatomy			5	5
Total	10	1	27	38

[a] One case combining adhesions and a functional ovarian cyst.

Ovarian cyst

Torsion of the ovary impedes proper evaluation of the ovarian cyst:
  – The ovary is increased in volume and appears obviously cystic.
  – Ischemia modifies the appearance and color of the ovarian surface; in addition, the cystic contents are always hemorrhagic.

Histologic examination is required. This means that the cyst is opened and a large piece of the wall excised, followed by careful inspection of the inner surface of the cyst. Ideally, a cystectomy should be performed unless the cyst is obviously functional. The diagnosis cannot be speculative; it must be certain. Because macroscopic diagnosis is unreliable, histology and follow-up are required. Homan published a study of 44 torsions, of which 26 involved ovarian cysts of unspecified histologic nature. This is a high number and, in itself, justifies second-look laparoscopy.

Tubal pathology (Fig. 17.12)

Ectopic pregnancy

Severe ischemia of the tube is also accompanied by an increase in volume, congestion of the wall, and sometimes some hemorrhagic fluid in the cul-de-sac. It is difficult to differentiate torsion of a normal tube from torsion of a tube containing an ectopic pregnancy. The differential diagnosis is based on clinical and biochemical information. If there is any doubt, salpingotomy is performed with rinsing-aspiration of the lumen for histologic examination. In one of our patients, this procedure was the only way to establish the diagnosis of ectopic pregnancy with certainty. In this situation, it is best not to use vasopressin analogues.

Distal tubal occlusion

Torsion makes differential diagnosis between hydrosalpinx and pyosalpinx difficult. History and physical are not very helpful. Leukocytosis and moderate fever also occur with torsion [2, 7, 8]. The endoscopic signs of infection are certainly more reliable: bilateral inflammation, the presence of purulent material, and agglutination of the involved organs. We consider that, when in doubt, salpingotomy should be performed, because drainage is required for optimal recovery of the tube.

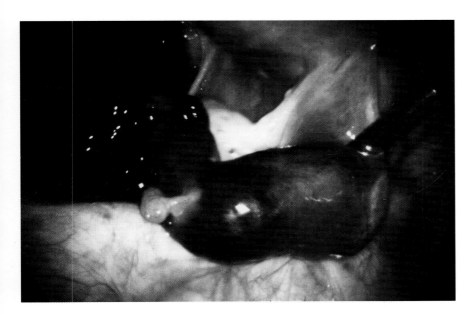

17.12 Torsion of an ectopic pregnancy. Only histologic examination can confirm or negate the diagnosis of ectopic pregnancy. A salpingotomy should be performed whenever a hematosalpinx is present.

Anatomic abnormalities

Lee [10] suggested that anomalies of insertion of the ovary are an etiologic factor. We have observed this in two cases: a long ovarian ligament and a short ovarian hilus (4 mm). In both cases, the ovary immediately returned to its torsed position, necessitating laparotomy for ovariopexy. Shortening of the ovarian ligament with a Yoon ring is a mistake, because the ligament necroses, leading to recurrence, as we have experienced.

Ovariopexy should be limited to cases of anatomic abnormality and should be bilateral if necessary. This procedure should not be routinely performed, because it is unnecessary [3, 5, 16]. Indeed, neither MacGowan, nor Way, nor Lee [12, 18, 10], nor we have seen recurrence if the adnexa were normal. Also, in the case of radical treatment of the torsion, it is rare to see recurrence on the contralateral side. Frequent episodes of acute pain prior to treatment of the torsion should not be the reason for "preventive surgery" on both ovarian ligaments, because in all these series such recurrent episodes of acute pain disappear with treatment of only the torsion (59 %, Lee; 25 %, Lomano; 53 %, Dunhihoo; 25 %, our data).

Inspection of the contralateral adnexa

Assessment of the contralateral tube should be routine, especially in the case of congenital abnormalities.

Radical treatment

Radical treatment is done by laparotomy in case of malignancy, irreversible lesions, torsion in the menopause, and torsion of the tube after ligation. A few other unusual conditions may also require radical treatment: ruptured extrauterine pregnancy, large ovarian cysts, or cysts having a suspicious appearance. Sometimes radical treatment is possible by laparoscopy; for example, salpingectomy for ectopic pregancy.

Unusual cases

In young girls [15, 16], diagnosis is extremely difficult but of the utmost importance, because untreated torsion is the main cause of adnexal autoamputation.

Results

The severity of the lesions (Table 17.1) correlates with the clinical picture. Torsion in the chronic group is never severe or irreversible. Acute torsion is a true emergency: 72 h later, the lesion is irreversible. The majority of etiologic factors can be treated conservatively: functional cysts of the ovary, paraovarian cysts, normal adnexa (29 in 38). All these factors serve to justify the use of laparoscopy and a conservative approach whenever possible. At the time of laparoscopy, detorsion was attempted 38 times. In 35 cases, it was successful; in the 3 others it caused the adnexa to abrupt because of the advanced stage of disease. (All 3 cases concerned torsed tubes only.) Our therapeutic approach is summarized in Table 17.3.

Laparotomy was required in 8 cases: 2 for necrosis of the adnexa, 5 for cystectomy of the ovary, 1 for ovariopexy. Treatment was completed at laparoscopy in 30 patients: conservatively in 24, radically in 6 (4 irreversible lesions, 1 salpingectomy for hydrosalpinx, 1 adnexectomy in menopause). The laparoscopic treatment is summarized in Table 17.4. The postoperative course was uneventful, without thromboembolic complications. Hospitalization lasted for 3 to 5 days. At second-look laparoscopy, conservative treatment of severe lesions has always been seen to result in complete recovery. Two patients were treated during the first trimester of pregnancy and successfully carried their pregnancies to term. Three other patients, one with a single adnexa, became pregnant after laparoscopic treatment of severe lesions.

TABLE 17.3 **Therapeutic plan for adnexal torsion**

		Minimal (N = 24)	Severe (N = 8)	Irreversible (N = 6)
Radical treatment	Laparoscopy	2	0	4
	Laparotomy	1	0	2
Conservative treatment	Laparoscopy	17	7	0
	Laparotomy	4	1	0

TABLE 17.4 **Endosurgical procedures**

Immediate	Detorsion	35
	Salpingectomy	3
Secondary	Adhesiolysis	2
	Puncture-biopsy of functional cyst	5
	Conservative treatment of EUP	1
	Pavaovarian cystectomy	10
	Ovarian cystectomy	2
	Oophorectomy	1
	Salpingectomy	5
	Ovariopexy with Yoon ring	2

Conclusion

The endoscopic approach to treatment of adnexal torsion is justified for attaining an accurate diagnosis and also, in many cases, for conservative surgical management. Conservative treatment is contraindicated in the presence of necrosis of the involved organs or of an organic tumor that is potentially malignant.

References

1. Azoury R.S., Chehab R.M., Mufarrij I.K., « The twisted adnexa; a clinical and pathological review », *Diagnostic Gynecology and Obstetrics*, 1980; 2 : 185-191.
2. Bernadus R.E., Van de Slikke J.W., Roex A.J.A., Dijkhuisen G.H., Stolk J.G., « Torsion of the fallopian tube: some consideration on its etiology », *Obstet. Gynecol.*, 1984; 64 : 675.
3. Beyth Y., Bar-On E., « Tubo ovarian auto amputation and infertility », *Obstet. Gynecol.*, 1979; 54 : 487.
4. Dellenbach P., « Malformations congénitales de la trompe », *In* « Oviducte et fertilité », Masson, 1979.
5. Dunnihoo D.R., Wolff J., « Bilateral torsion of the adnexa: a case report and review of the literature », *Obstet. Gynecol.*, 1984; 55 : 64.
6. Evans J.P., « Torsion of the normal uterine adnexa in premenarchal girls », *Journal of Pediatric Surgery*, 1978; 13: 195.
7. Filtenborg T.A., Hertz J.B., « Case report: torsion of the fallopian tube », *Europ. J. Obstet. Gynecol. Reprod. Biol.*, 1981; 12 : 177-181.
8. Hurwitz A., Milwidsky A., Yagel S., Adoni A., « Early unwinding of torsion of an ovarian cyst as a result of hyperstimulation syndrome », *Fertil. Steril.*, 1983; 40 : 393.
9. James D.F., Barber H.R.K., Graber E.A., « Torsion of uterine adnexa in children. Report of three cases », *Obstet. Gynecol.*, 1970; 35 : 226.
10. Lee R.A., Welch J.S., « Torsion of the uterine adnexa », *Am. J. Obstet. Gynecol.*, 1967; 97 : 974.
11. Lomano J.M., Trelford J.D., Ullery J.C., « Torsion of the uterine adnexa causing an acute abdomen », *Obstet. Gynecol.*, 1970; 35 : 221.
12. MacGowan L., « Torsion of cystic or diseased adnexal tissue », *Am. J. Obstet. Gynecol.*, 1964; 88 : 135.
13. Mage G., Michelot J., Lagoutte M., Lagarde N., Gaillard G., Bruhat M.A., « Autogreffe ovarienne chez la lapine. Etude expérimentale », *J. Gynecol. Obstet. Biol. Reprod.*, 1979; 8 : 483.
14. Mage G., Canis M., Manhes H., Pouly J.L., Wattiez A., Bruhat M.A., « Laparoscopic management of adnexal cystic tumors », *J. of Reproductive Medecine* (à paraître).
15. Manhes H., Canis M., Mage G., Pouly J.L., Bruhat M.A., « Place de la cœlioscopie dans le diagnostic et le traitement des torsions d'annexes », *J. Gynecol. Obstet. Biol. Reprod.*, 1984; 13 : 825.
16. Moravec W.D., Angerman N.S., Reale F.R., Hajj S.N., « Torsion of the uterine adnexa: a clinicopathologic correlation », *Int. J. Gynecol Obstet.*, 1980; 18 : 7.
17. Sebastian J.A., Baker R.L., Cordray D., « Asymptomatic infarction and separation of the ovary and distal uterine tube », *Obstet. Gynecol.*, 1931; 41 : 531.
18. Way S., « Ovarian cystectomy of twisted cysts », *Lancet*, 1946; 2 : 47.

18

Laparoscopic hysterectomy

Hysterectomy remains one of the more common procedures performed in gynecology. Recent breakthroughs in operative hysteroscopy have eliminated some of the indications, such as submucous myoma. Exeresis of the uterus remains the treatment of choice for conditions such as precancerous and cancerous lesions of the uterus and cervix. Lymphadenectomy may be performed during the same session.

Abdominal hysterectomy can be achieved through a vertical or transverse incision (Mouchel, Pfannenstiel). Access to the uterus and adnexa is quite easy in this fashion. In addition, the surgery can be expanded to include the parametria and lymphatic chains. Surgical correction of prolapse or stress urinary incontinence is equally feasible.

Hysterectomy may also be performed by the vaginal route. In this case, as opposed to abdominal surgery, however, the bulk of the uterus is a significant limiting factor. The size of the uterus is not a contraindication per se. However, the operator should observe some limits. When traction is applied to the cervix, one expects mobilization 3 cm or more.

Adnexal surgery is a difficult task through vaginal access, and lymph node dissection is out of the question. Vaginal hysterectomy can be extended to include the parametria, according to the technique described by Shauta [3]. The vaginal approach is thus not suitable when adnexal surgery or lymph node surgery is required. On the other hand, the advantages of vaginal surgery are reduced postoperative morbidity, avoidance of an abdominal scar, and the possibility of performing concomitant surgery for prolapse and stress incontinence.

In this chapter we discuss laparoscopic hysterectomy as compared to the established procedures.

Procedure

Positioning of the patient

The patient is draped so as to permit access to the vagina. She lies in the dorsal decubitus position with the legs slightly flexed and abducted to form a 45° angle. This is the position favored by surgeons for abdominoperineal procedures. A Foley catheter is placed. Insertion of a uterus manipulator is paramount, because it will allow increased exposure during the procedure. We place a smooth curette attached to two cervical tenaculums into the uterine cavity. In this way, risk of perforation is minimal, and the instrument is long enough that the uterus can be pushed up to the umbilicus. In addition, a rotating motion can be applied to the uterus. Trendelenburg position is reduced to a minimum as long as the bowel remains above the promontory. A good bowel preparation facilitates the latter.

Three suprapubic 5-mm trocars are placed for insertion of ancillary instruments. The lateral trocars are placed two to three finger breadths above the pubis, either at the outer limits of the "safety triangle" or lateral to the epigastic vessels. The median trocar is placed two to three finger breadths above the level of the other two.

Materials

Video equipment is mandatory. Through the ancillary trocars, four types of instruments can be introduced: scissors, graspers, rinsing/aspiration probe, and bipolar forceps. If clips are used, one of the ancillary trocars should be 10 mm in diameter.

Successive steps

Coagulation and transection of the infundibulopelvic ligaments

Bipolar coagulation is used in several successive bites. The desiccated zone should blanch over an area of at least 1 cm. The incision with scissors is made at a right angle.

Bladder flap preparation

The uterus is pushed up and cephalad to stretch the anterior peritoneal leaf. A grasper is applied to the bladder flap or the round ligament and the peritoneum incised with scissors down to the vaginal wall. If difficulties are encountered, this part of the dissection can be finished after the broad ligament and uterine arteries are transected, which increases the mobility of the uterus and thereby the exposure.

Desiccation and section of the uterine arteries

This is achieved with bipolar coagulation, possibly in association with a clip. The vessels should be isolated prior to section and coagulation performed at a right angle, close to the uterus. The operator should desiccate the vessel for at least 1 cm and proceed from outside to inside and from below upward.

Desiccation and section of cardinal ligaments

This is also done with bipolar coagulation, as close as possible to the uterus, either intra- or extrafascially. This process of successive cutting and coagulation is continued until the lateral vaginal wall is reached. A sponge pushed up into the lateral vaginal fornix facilitates orientation.

Desiccation and section of the sacrouterine ligaments

First the posterior peritoneum is incised. Then the ligaments are desiccated and sectioned at a level flush with the uterus. This can be done prior to or following section of the cardinal ligaments. It may be necessary to increase the Trendelenburg temporarily.

Incision of the vaginal wall

This is done at the anterior fornix with scissors or with the monopolar needle. Again, a sponge pushed up the vagina facilitates orientation. This will also retard the loss of pneumoperitoneum.

Uterine extraction and vaginal closure

This part of the procedure encompasses the following:
- Incision of the vaginal wall, which is marked with sutures to facilitate closure
  - Extraction of the uterus
  - Closure of the vaginal cuff

Peritoneal lavage

Hemostasis is assured laparoscopically and the pelvic cavity is thoroughly rinsed. The raw area may be sprayed with biocompatible glue to prevent adhesion formation. (As of early 1991, this substance was not yet available in the United States.)

Variations

According to the extent of the procedure performed laparoscopically, there are three types of hysterectomy:

Type 1: The endosurgery is limited to the adnexa.

Type 2: The procedure is extended to include desiccation and section of the uterine vessels. The cardinal ligaments and uterosacral ligaments are ligated vaginally.

Type 3: The procedure in its entirety is carried out endoscopically, including opening of the vaginal wall.

Type 1 can be considered only as a prelude to vaginal hysterectomy, whereas types 2 and 3 are truly endosurgical hysterectomies.

Concomitant procedures

Adhesiolysis: Adhesiolysis may be required to increase access to the uterus and adnexa. For more details, see Chapter 9.

Lymphadenectomy: A lymphadenectomy, when indicated, is performed before the vagina is opened, according to the technique described in Chapter 19.

Radical hysterectomy: When required, hysterectomy can be done in such a way as to include the parametria and ligation of the uterine artery at the level of the ureter.

Patient selection

Between September 1989 and December 1990, 36 patients underwent either partial or complete endosurgical hysterectomy. The indications and types of surgery are reported in Tables 18.1 and 18.2, respectively.

TABLE 18.1 **Preoperative diagnosis**

Therapy-resistant abnormal uterine bleeding	13
Uterus myomatosus (no abnormal bleeding)	8
Precancerous lesions	7
Cervical and endometrial malignancies	8
Total	36

TABLE 18.2 **Type of surgery**

Simple hysterectomy	28
Hysterectomy and lymphadenectomy	4
Extended hysterectomy	1
Extended hysterectomy and lymphadenectomy	3
Total	36

Results

Twenty-seven of 36 (75%) surgical procedures were completed laparoscopically. Nine (25%) were converted to laparotomy because of difficulties in establishing hemostasis (6 cases) and in order to locate anatomic landmarks (3 cases). Problems with hemostasis occurred four times at the level of the uterine artery and twice at the level of the cardinal ligaments.

Laparotomy was performed prior to serious blood loss, and tranfusion was not required. The other patients presented with either a large uterus (1 case) blocking access to the vascular pedicle, a myoma of the broad ligament (1 case), and a hypertrophied cervix that impeded dissection of the ureter. Failure in relation to indication and type of intervention are presented in Table 18.3. Five of the six patients were scheduled to undergo simple hysterectomy. No bladder or bowel injury occurred during these procedures. Postoperative recovery was uncomplicated: no delayed hemorrhage occurred as a result of these procedures. One patient underwent laparoscopy on the second postoperative day for what was thought to be a subocclusion. No pathology was found, and it is assumed that this patient suffered a delayed return to normal transit. The need for analgesia in the immediate postoperative period is lower, compared to abdominal hysterectomy. Bowel function resumed within 36 h of surgery. Intravenous pyelography performed on day 10 in the 3 cases of radical hysterectomy was within normal limits. Blood transfusion was not required in any case. The average hospital stay for the entire patient population was 5 to 6 days. Those patients undergoing simple hysterectomy stayed only 4 days. (Note from translator: Hospital stay in Europe is on the average 3 to 4 times longer than in the United States.)

TABLE 18.3 **Failed endosurgical procedure (laparotomy required)**

As a function of the type of surgery	
Simple hysterectomy	8
Hysterectomy and lymphadenectomy	0
Extended hysterectomy	0
Extended hysterectomy and lymphadenectomy	1
Total	9
As a function of preoperative diagnosis	
Thereapy-resistant abnormal uterine bleeding	5
Uterus myomatosus (no abnormal bleeding)	3
Precancerous lesions	0
Cervical and endometrial malignancies	1
Total	9

Discussion

This preliminary data indicate that experienced endosurgeons can perform a hysterectomy safely. Reich reported the first case in 1988 [1]. Using bipolar desiccation we encountered no difficulties in establishing hemostasis at the level of the ovarian or infundibulopelvic ligament.

We experienced an equally successful outcome in adnexal surgery. The following should be emphasized, however: (1) The ureter should be located prior to section of the infundibulopelvic ligament and (2) when the adnexa are left in situ, section of the pedicles is best performed as far away from the uterus as possible, to avoid significant back bleeding.

The six failures we experienced during dissection of the uterine or cardinal pedicles could be dealt with quite simply at laparotomy. These failures occurred, of course, early on. At the level of the uterine pedicle, there is a tendency to coagulate too far from the uterus from fear of compromising the ureter. Coagulation is then incomplete. Our first failure happened during removal of the uterus, at which time the uterine stump avulsed. We suspect that the desiccation had been insufficient. In addition, because of the angle of approach of the ancillary instruments, the surgeon has a tendency to cut the pedicles parallel to the lateral uterine border. When the cardinal ligaments are transected, it is wise to obtain a panoramic view in order to ensure that sectioning is done close to the cervix. The lateral vaginal fornices should be reached. Early in our experience, we had to place clamps on the lateral vaginal wall to ensure hemostasis.

The main limitation remains the size of the uterus. The largest uterus we removed endosurgically approximated the size of a 12-week pregnancy. The presence of adhesions is not a contraindication, but it certainly prolongs the surgery.

Compared to abdominal surgery, endosurgery offers all the advantages of laparoscopy: less trauma, shorter hospital stay, and reduced costs. A measure of the latter is provided by the lessened need for analgesics postoperatively. In addition, bowel function is recovered within 36 h. The absence of a large scar allows early ambulation, which is a major advantage for elderly patients.

Vaginal surgery offers similar advantages. However, the endosurgical access allows for optimal exploration of the pelvic cavity and adnexa. This is an important aspect in the presence of endometrial cancer or ovarian pathology. In addition, lymph node dissection can be performed at the same time. Obviously, some patients with a history of endometriosis or uterine antefixation will benefit from the laparoscopic approach. This procedure will find its place next to other endosurgical and vaginal procedures for treatment of benign uterine pathology. In many cases, the problems caused by enlargement of the uterus can be obviated by the use of luteinizing hormone releasing hormone (LH-RH) analogues.

Regarding malignant conditions, conclusions should be drawn more carefully. Endosurgical treatment of the obese, hypertensive, elderly patient with endometrial cancer, stage 1a, is appealing. The hospital stay and also the risk for thromboembolic accidents are reduced because the patient is bedridden for only a short time. The study of larger series of patients is required, however, before conclusions can be drawn, especially with regard to the increased challenge from changes in parameters related to anesthesia. In cancer of the cervix, the indications for surgery are limited to stages T1a2 and T1b (low volume). In the latter case, surgical treatment is preceded by brachytherapy.

Endosurgical hysterectomy as a technique is still in the early phase of evaluation. This intervention should, therefore, be performed only be experienced endoscopists. Moreover, the new equipment needed is still only in the prototype stage. Improved equipment will certainly be of help to everyone who performs endosurgical procedures.

References

1. Reich H., « Laparoscopic hysterectomy », *J. Gynecol. Surg.*, 1989; 5 : 2.
2. Mage G., Canis M., Wattiez A., Pouly J.L., Bruhat M.A., « Hysterectomie et cœlioscopie », *J. Gynecol. Obstet. Biol. Reprod.*, 1990; 19 : 573-576.
3. Schauta F., « Die enveiterte vaginale totale extirpation der uterus bei kollumcarzinom », Wein. Leipzig, J. Safar. 1908.

19

Laparoscopic lymphadenectomy

The staging of a malignancy is invaluable for determining the prognosis. Invasion of the lymph nodes is one of the more important factors in deciding the course of treatment. Noninvasive techniques for evaluating nodal status such as lymphography and CT scan are burdened by false-positive and false-negative readings. The specificity of these methods does not exceed 85 % at best [1–3]. The use of magnetic resonance imaging is fairly recent, and apparently specificity is only 65 % for cancer of the cervix. Guided needle aspiration techniques are of interest because they provide a histologic sample. However, only a positive result is of any value.

The lack of specificity of the above methods has led to the development of other techniques that allow histologic evaluation of tissue blocks. This approach is the only one resulting in a definitive answer regarding nodal status. The techniques described are retroperitoneoscopy [2, 4] and laparoscopy [5].

Laparoscopy seems to us to be the preferred method and can be integrated in the therapeutic plan for cancer of the cervix [5]. Survival is directly related to nodal status. Treatment plans can be set up for patients with positive nodes and those whose nodes are negative. The results obtained with this method are histologic and definite.

Review of the anatomy

Lymphatic drainage varies widely from one individual to another. In France, it is customary to use the classification of Cune and Marcille, which divides the pelvic lymph nodes into the common, external, and internal iliac groups.

The external iliac group runs along the external iliac vessels. According to Leveuf and Godard, these nodes are the most important group and can be subdivided into three branches, which are situated in the parametrium lateral to the ureter. These three groups encompass (1) the external branch, also called the *arterial, or lateral, branch*; (2) the intermediate branch, also called the *prevenous, or middle, branch*; and (3) the internal branch, also called the *obturator, or infravenous, branch* (Fig. 19.1.)

The external branch

This branch is inconsistent. It runs between the external iliac artery medially and the psoas muscle laterally. The most consistent node is the one located distally, which is called the *external retrocrural node*. This node lies behind the inguinal ligament.

The intermediate branch

This is the most inconsistent of all three branches. It is located between the external iliac artery and vein. The most distal node, the middle crural node, as

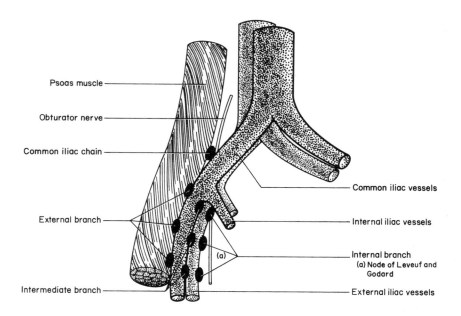

Psoas muscle

Obturator nerve

Common iliac chain

External branch

Intermediate branch

Common iliac vessels

Internal iliac vessels

Internal branch
(a) Node of Leveuf and
Godard

External iliac vessels

well as the node situated at the level of the node of Leveuf and Godard, is not always present. The most consistent node is the one located at the bifurcation, which also communicates with the common iliac lymphatic chain.

The internal branch

This is the most important branch and is located between the obturator nerve and the external iliac vein. The internal retrocrural node drains the deep inguinal region. This node is consistent and communicates with the node of Leveuf and Godard, which is equally consistent. The third node, located at the level of the bifurcation, if present, communicates with the common iliac chain.

Procedure

The initial steps are similar to those for any other laparoscopy for pelvic surgery. Three suprapubic trocars are required. A Hegar probe is inserted into the uterus for manipulation. If a hysterectomy is to be performed in the same session, other factors intervene, as explained in Chapter 18. First the abdominal cavity is inspected carefully. Then the uterus is placed in anteversion and pushed to the side opposite to the dissection (to the left for dissection of the right side and to the right for dissection of the left side). The first step is to identify the umbilical ligament. The ligament is grasped in its anterior portion. Traction will facilitate identification of the lower portion of the ligament, between the round ligament and the infundibulopelvic ligament. The peritoneum is then incised immediately lateral to the ligament and parallel to it. The umbilical ligament can then be grasped at the level of the iliac vessels and dissection can be carried out, with scissors or graspers, immediately lateral to the ligament. Then follows dissection of the medial aspect of the nodal chain. The nodal tissue is then freed from the undersurface of the iliac vein until the pelvic side wall is reached. The lower border of the dissection is formed by the obturator nerve. The lymphatic chain is coagulated with bipolar forceps, transected at the level of the inguinal ligament, and grasped with claw forceps. By holding the string of tissue up, the freeing of the obturator nerve from the nodes will be facilitated. The proximal end of the dissection, at the level of the iliac bifurcation, is the most difficult part of the procedure, requiring diligence and restraint.

Small vessels and vascular pedicles must be coagulated with bipolar forceps prior to section. Even a small amount of bleeding will obscure the operators' view, because the intervention is performed in a narrow space. When dissection is completed, the sample is removed with a three-pronged forceps or a 10-mm cup forceps. One of the suprapubic ports must be changed from 5 to 10 mm in diameter. The pelvic cavity is then thoroughly rinsed with a physiologic solution to check hemostasis. The peritoneal incisions are left open so that lymphatic drainage can occur through the abdominal cavity, thereby avoiding formation of a lymphocele.

Results

From November 1989 until November 1990, 13 patients underwent laparoscopic lymphadenectomy. The age of the patients varied from 30 to 72. The patients can be subdivided into three groups: cancer of the cervix (N = 8), cancer of the endometrium (N = 4), and cancer of the vulva and clitoris (N = 1) (see Table 19.1).

No intraoperative complications occurred. The duration of surgery was less than 1 h. An average of 4.4 and 4.3 lymph nodes were removed from the right and left sides, respectively, with ranges from 1 to 10 on the right and 1 to 8 on the left. No node was found to be positive in this limited series. When laparoscopic surgery for endometrial cancer was performed, a hysterectomy was performed during the same session.

TABLE 19.1 **Patients for laparoscopic lymphadenectomy**

Type and staging	Number of cases
Cervix 1a2 (diagnosis by cone biopsy)	4
Cervix 1b	4
Endometrium 1a	4
Vulva	1

Discussion

Laparoscopic lymphadenectomy is a reliable diagnostic intervention. The specimen thus obtained is adequate and viewing of the anatomic spaces is actually better at laparoscopy than at laparotomy.

What are the indications for this procedure?

Adenocarcinoma of the endometrium. A hysterectomy, either vaginal or endosurgical, can be performed at the same time for stages 1a and 1b. The avoidance of laparotomy in this elderly patient population is an obvious advantage. However, one should investigate whether the patient's cardiovascular condition will tolerate the burden of laparoscopy.

Squamous cell carcinoma of the cervix. Laparoscopic lymphadenectomy may become part of the workup of the patient prior to treatment of the malignancy. It has been shown that if the external iliac lymph nodes are negative, invasion of the common iliac or aortic nodes is less than 1 % ("skip nodes"). Laparoscopic pelvic node sampling is then acceptably reliable. A therapeutic plan for treatment of the cervical malignancy can therefore be tailored to the histologic rather than the clinical staging of the disease. One may anticipate that such a plan will, in the future, simplify the treatment dilemma and reduce the cost and morbidity associated with treatment of this condition.

References

1. Bartel M., « Die Retroperitoneoskopie: Eine endoskopische Methode zur Inspektion und biologischen Untersuchung des retroperitonealen Raumes », *Zentralbl. Chir.*, 1969; 74 : 337-383.
2. Wurtz H., Luch H., « Reflexions a propos de la retroperitoneoscopie operatoire en gynecologie », *Presse Med.*, 1987; 16 : 1865.
3. Hacher N.F., Berek J.S., « Surgical staging of cervical cancer », In E.A. Survit, O.S. Alberts (Eds.), *Cervix Cancer*. Boston, Martinus Nijhoff.
4. Dargent D., Salvat J., « L'Envahissement ganglionnaire pelvien ». New York, McGraw-Hill, 1989.
5. Querleu D., Leblan E., Cartelain B., « Lymphadenectomie pelvienne sous controle cœlioscopique », *J. Gyn. Obstet. Biol. Reprod.*, 1990; 19 : 576.

Index

Achevé d'imprimer en octobre 1991
par SOULISSE et CASSEGRAIN (Niort)
pour MEDSI/McGRAW-HILL
N° d'imprimeur : 2952
Dépôt légal : octobre 1991

Imprimé en France